Yoga

A Simple Guide to Looking & Feeling Better With Yoga Poses for Beginners

(Relieve Yourself of Back, Neck and Whole Body Pain)

Leslie Brown

Published by Rob Miles

Leslie Brown

All Rights Reserved

Yoga: A Simple Guide to Looking & Feeling Better With Yoga Poses for Beginners (Relieve Yourself of Back, Neck and Whole Body Pain)

ISBN 978-1-989990-54-4

Legal & Disclaimer

The information contained in this book is not designed to replace or take the place of any form of medicine or professional medical advice. The information in this book has been provided for educational and entertainment purposes only.

The information contained in this book has been compiled from sources deemed reliable, and it is accurate to the best of the Author's knowledge; however, the Author cannot guarantee its accuracy and validity and cannot be held liable for any errors or omissions. Changes are periodically made to this book. You must consult your doctor or get professional medical advice before using any of the suggested remedies, techniques, or information in this book.

Table of Contents

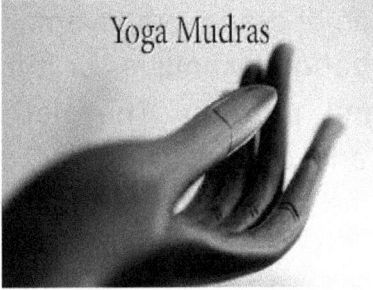

Yoga Mudras

The Sanskrit word mudra is translated as 'gesture' or 'attitude.' Mudras can be described as psychic, emotional, devotional and aesthetic gestures or attitudes. Yogis have experienced mudras as attitudes of energy flow, intended to link individual pranic force with universal or cosmic force. The Kularnava Tantra traces the word mudra to the root mud meaning 'delight' or 'pleasure' and dravay, the causal form of dru which means 'to draw forth.' Mudra is also defined as a 'seal,' 'short-cut' or 'circuit by-pass.'

1

Mudras are a combination of subtle physical movements which alter mood, attitude and perception, and which deepen awareness and concentration. A mudra may involve the whole body in a combination of asana, pranayama, bandha and visualization techniques or it may be a simple hand position. The Hatha Yoga Pradipika and other yogic texts consider mudra to be a yoganda, an independent branch of yoga, requiring a very subtle awareness. Mudras are introduced after some proficiency has been attained in asana, pranayama and bandha, and gross blockages have been removed.

Mudras have been described in various texts from antiquity to the present day in order to preserve them for posterity. However, such references were never detailed or clearly delineated as these techniques were not intended to be learned from a book. Practical instruction from a guru was always considered to be a necessary requisite before attempting them. Mudras are higher practices which lead to awakening of the pranas, chakras and kundalini, and which can bestow major siddhis, psychic powers, on the advanced practitioner.

CHAPTER 1: THE HISTORY OF YOGA

Yoga has a very interesting and varied history. When you look back through the history, the point that stands out the most is where yoga and Buddhism come into touch with each other. People in India used yoga over 5000 years ago, but for me, the relevant history that gives me the biggest clue as to why it is still followed today is the story of the first Buddha. His idea was to go into meditation and seek out the reasons why mankind suffers so much. Although I could dwell on the history of yoga from many different perspectives, it is this one that I believe will convince you more than any other. During his time meditating through yoga meditation, the first Buddha actually came up with the answer to his question on mankind's suffering and found that most of it was caused by man himself.

By stepping into the future and worrying about it and using lessons from the past to make barriers against personal growth, what people did was restrict themselves. He then wrote the text which is respected by Buddhists and which actually gives them guidelines to live their lives by. Although people associate this with religion, Buddhism is actually a philosophy, rather than a religion.

The Bhagavad-Gîtâ, which is one of the most famous texts on yoga came before this time and can probably be classified as pre-classical. This text is still referred to today and forms the basis for many yoga practitioners' beliefs, in that it teaches those who practice yoga to put aside the negative aspects of humanity such as ego and to learn wisdom. While different to the Buddhist interpretation of yoga, what makes me so curious about both of these different ways of thinking is that they achieve one and the same thing – harmony and understanding. When you think that one event, i.e. the writing of the Bhagavad-Gita was approximately 500 years before Christ and the other event –

the meditation of the original Buddha –in about 430 were years apart, the similarity of what both types of yoga encompass is what people need to bear in mind. One type touches on the subject of karma, while the other concentrates on oneness.

From these humble beginnings came the Four Noble Truths and the Eightfold Path that is followed by Buddhists today in an effort to reach that place which presents them with perfection. When you watch Buddhist monks during meditation, you cannot help but be drawn into the feeling of overall peace and tranquility that they appear to be able to achieve and all of this is by following the written works of the first Buddha. Thus, the history is relevant because it forms part of today's yoga meditation and is thus not something that can be discounted as past history. Its history that is alive and very much kicking in a world perhaps a distance from where you are living and reading this book, but its relevance to you is every bit as important today as it was at the time that it was written.

Although you may be wondering where this is going when all you wanted was to look for a way to lose weight and heal your body and even invigorate your mind, I feel it is of significance because unless you know where yoga comes from, you can't fully appreciate its longevity. Things that work last. People have been practicing yoga for more than 5000 years and it may only have been recently that you have started to think of trying this as a treatment to help you get through the stresses and strains of today's world, although while you were an infant, Buddhist monks were practicing this and taking the Eightfold path that they still see as relevant today. The fulfillment of your life's journey can begin here.

Interestingly enough, when yoga was introduced to the western world in Chicago at the turn of the 20th century, it wowed those that listened to the talks and who found what they heard to be enlightening. Hatha yoga became more and more accepted in the western world at this time and has since gained much popularity with young and old alike as being a way of life that can be embraced by anyone.

Of course, the history is much deeper than these two pages have described, but the purpose of this book is to pass to you the different methods rather than to delve into an in depth history. Suffice it to say that there is enough history to make it a potential to add to your life, a potential that has been found to be very powerful indeed and which will help you to develop your spiritual self as well as making the most of your physical self.

Holistic approaches are becoming more and more recognized as being able to provide more for the individual than the alternatives offered by modern science and it's small wonder. Go through the pages of YouTube and listen to lectures on yoga and you will find that there's a convincing argument for the benefits of yoga to those trying to improve their lifestyles and their actual approach to life. It's the same now – in this moment – that opportunity sits and awaits you. This book is written in as simple a manner as possible to include as much information for the uninitiated as is seen as relevant to help people to gain better health, happiness and self-realization than they thought possible, which is what the roots of yoga is all about.

CHAPTER 2: WHY FOOT YOGA?

The Merriam-Webster dictionary defines yoga as a system of physical postures, breathing techniques, and sometimes meditation derived from Yoga but often practiced independently especially in Western cultures to promote physical and emotional well-being.

Yoga is so much more than putting your body in complex positions that look impossible at first.Yoga is also about your breath, your thoughts and how you feel in any given moment.It's about getting to know your body and it's also about noticing when something isn't working for your body.It's as much about awareness as is about taking action to make a change.

Without awareness of what is happening right now, there can be no change.You must first notice what is before you can change to what you want.

This combination of awareness and change is what I've tried to put together in this e-book.My goal is to help you to become aware of what's happening in your feet so that you can begin to feel better.Accept that your feet ache or hurt sometimes and that this affects the rest of your body and mind.Accept that you can make a difference with your feet.It will take a little time and effort but the results will be worth it.

Self-care starts with your feet How much do you think about your feet?I'm willing to bet that until they start hurting, you don't think too much about them.They get you where you need to go every day, support you as you stand around to work, cook, or chat, and they take you to fun places like the park or the beach. Your feet are responsible for getting you from one place to another throughout the day, yet you don't spend too much time taking care of them.With all that your feet do for you, why not do something for them?

Now, I don't mean go and get a pedicure.Sure, having your toes freshly painted can make your feet look nice, but it doesn't do anything for the structure of your foot.What about a massage or some foot exercises?What about soaking them in Epsom salts after a long day?There are so many actions that we can take to make our feet healthier. I've often heard that if your feet hurt, then the rest of your body hurts. Does that sound familiar to you?

Think back to a time when you spent many hours on your feet.They were probably tired and/or aching. This led to the rest of you being tired and, most likely, something else in your body hurt too.Taking care of your feet can reverse this.After all, healthier feet feel better and will take you much farther in life.This e-book will outline several actions that you can take in order to create happier, healthier feet.Your feet will thank you for taking better care of them by feeling better than they have in a long time.Once

your feet feel better, then the rest of you
will feel better too!

CHAPTER 3: WHAT IS YOGA?

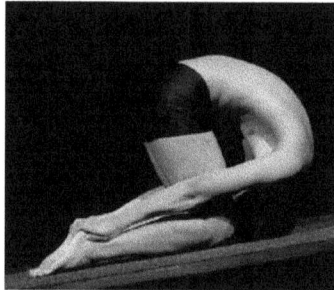

The origins of yoga are firmly steeped in history. It is a gentle age old practice that works on the body, mind and spirit in a holistic manner. It was formed in India over 5000 years ago, although in those times, yoga was very different to the practice of today. The classical period is defined by the Yoga Sutras which is the first presentation of yoga, written in the 2nd century, describing Raja Yoga – and this is often denoted as classical yoga.

Although the teachings of yoga are spiritual, in the Western world, those interested in studying yoga will choose whether they wish to focus more on the physical application of yoga or to include the spiritual elements. Some yoga students care little for the history, while for others, there is a greater appreciation of how yoga has evolved through time.

This course focuses on the postures, the benefits and the principles of each pose as well as the correct alignment which will aid your student's progress and enable you to teach in a proficient manner. This is a Hatha yoga course so has a strong connection with the physical element of yoga but it is important to note that there are many different styles including:

Ashtanga yoga Iyengar yoga Power yoga Anusara yoga etc.

Hatha yoga-utilises every aspect of self:

Mentally
Emotionally Physically

The postures are very powerful irrespective of the students ' current stage of flexibility when first joining your class. Even those students who can only move a little, will find that their body embraces the gentleness of the movements and will gradually relax into the postures. Always take the time to find out more about your students – especially when considering any health implications.

Yoga means union and Hatha is derived from ha (sun) and tha (moon) and it signifies both consciousness and the life force. Dedicated Hatha yogis discovered through their meticulous practice of each posture (asana) that it is possible to obtain a beautiful balance of mind, body and spirit. This is the true reward of yoga.

Students' begin to recognise the potential to cleanse their bodies, to improve circulation and to revitalise their internal organs while toning muscles, strengthening joints and easing the nerves. They discovered that yoga affects every aspect of the body's ability to heal and function in an optimal manner. Some of the Hatha yoga styles are known as being pure forms in that they have a direct lineage to India. Other styles may have developed substantially over the years and now resemble little to those traditional forms of Hatha yoga. In recent decades, it could be said that yoga has changed and developed far more than throughout its long history. Some teachers stick rigidly to the original teachings while others are prepared to adapt sessions and evolve.

As a teacher you will need to know a great deal about yoga, not just in terms of style and postural benefits but as to the deep roots of your teaching practice. It is important to be dedicated to the practice of yoga and to believe whole-heartedly in this simple practice. By living the yogic way, you will feel more confident when teaching your students.

Let's look at just some of the yoga styles:
Iyengar yoga

B.K.S Iyengar was born in 1918 and he bought this style of yoga into great popularity. In his early years, he was often less physically able than many of his students and as a result, began to experiment with modifications to the postures and to use props. These methods of adaptation are linked only to Iyengar yoga and his very detailed sets of instructions which included information on alignment within each pose has changed Hatha yoga.

He believed that a posture was only achieved providing the whole of the body was positioned correctly and also, felt that the full benefits could only be achieved once the student was comfortable in the extended posture. By using props, students were able to achieve an extended pose suitable for their level of flexibility and therefore, benefits could be realised much earlier. Nowadays, there are bolsters, blankets, straps and blocks designed to help students with stability in difficult postures and to help them to adjust their body accordingly. While Hatha yoga concentrates on the physical aspects, it does not use the props of Iyengar yoga.

Bikram yoga

Bikram Choudhury is the leading teacher of Bikram yoga and has many dedicated followers. It is also known as Hot yoga. Choudhury developed a 26 pose and 2 breathing exercise routine style after meticulously researching yoga. It is a very specific style of yoga where the room temperature for each class is set at 105°F. Students have to complete the 26 poses twice within a set sequence. The sets do not include arm balances or inversions. Choudhury believes that his style of yoga is the true style. Certainly, by stretching in a heated room, the ability to stretch is greater than would be possible normally. However, the potential to extend too far is a cause for concern.

Integral yoga

Integral yoga integrates many different aspects of yoga into the one style-although to confuse the matter, there are two separate Integral yoga styles. One is founded by Ramaswamy Satchidananda and the other by Aurobindo Akroyd Ghosh. Both established large followings and networks of teaching centres.

Both styles go far beyond the physical practice of postures and include meditation, devotion, deep study, and mantras as they integrate all the major branches of yoga. Satchidananda's approach was that postures along with breath control, cleansing practices and relaxation would strengthen the body and mind. His classes were gentle and offered breath-work, chanting and meditation.

Ananda yoga

This is based on the teachings of Paramahansa Yogananda who was the founder of the Self Realisation Fellowship. The purpose of practising asana and pranayama is to awaken the life force and to control the flow of energy within leading to an increased awareness and uplifted consciousness. It differs from other Hatha yoga styles in that it has energiser exercises and affirmations. There are 39 energy techniques and the affirmations are practiced silently during the pose. There is great emphasis on correct alignment and on being relaxed in the midst of the postures.

Ashtanga Vinyasa yoga

Within the yoga sutras, the term Ashtanga means eight limbs but it is also the name of the yoga taught by Pattabhi Jois of Mysore and it is practiced on a worldwide scale. Although known mainly as Ashtanga, the full name is Ashtanga Vinyasa Yoga. This method is firmly grounded in the Yoga Sutras. Asanas are grouped into a six series - which makes a set sequence. It also teaches philosophy, mudra, bandha, drishti and vinyasa. Students are taught in the Mysore style and each student individually moves through the sequence on their own so that the teacher can give personalised guidance. Students new to Hatha yoga often find this style very difficult.

Kundalini yoga

Kundalini yoga may seem a distant variation of traditional Hatha yoga because there is less focus on the physical postures but greater attention on meditation, chanting and the breath. This style was brought to the West in 1969 and the Kundalini techniques used to be practised in secret because they were considered both powerful and dangerous. The aim is to use a variety of techniques so as to move energy through the chakras by way of mantras, mudras, pranayama's and different postures. It is known as an intense practice as the arms are often held aloft through extended periods, there are also extended periods of meditation and the breath too is extended.

Sivananda yoga

Swami Sivananda who died in 1963 had a tremendous influence on Hatha yoga and this style starts with relaxation in the corpse pose (Savasana) and follows with 12 asana before resting in Savasana and then utilising full yogic breathing. There are also 3 methods of relaxation using auto suggestion to ensure the individual falls into a deep state of relaxation.

Some yoga styles are a fusion of others and even include other exercise systems such as martial arts. While there are other styles of Hatha yoga, it's important to understand that although some styles

state there is a direct line to the origins of yoga, it is clear to see that there is often a fusion of styles too and perhaps more so in the Western world. In fact, many styles have drawn insights from dance, martial arts, gymnastics as well as other yoga styles.

To study and to become fully proficient in some of the styles mentioned, you will need to take your teacher training further and to study at specific schools - often for many years before teacher certification is provided.

This course teaches basic Hatha yoga qualifying you to teach and to then choose the style of your choice as you wish and to develop further within teacher training if you so choose.

Being a yoga teacher means being aware of students needs and you may find that limiting yourself to one style does not provide sufficient flexibility to encompass all of their needs. You may need to offer variations and modify certain postures, you may even suggest students learn alternate styles of yoga or have to choose how to adapt your own style of teaching. But the most important aspect of being a yoga teacher is your understanding of the techniques, the postures and alignment and being dedicated to help with your students' progression.

Sanskrit is the language of India's ancient texts and this gave rise to both the literature and technique of the yoga practice of today. Each yoga pose, 'asana' has a Sanskrit name which can

be used in addition to the name in English.

Self-Study Assessments

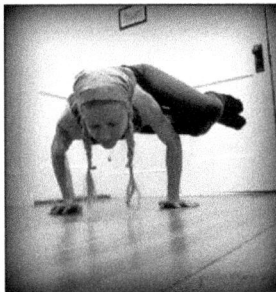

Task:
Consider why you wish to train as a teacher of yoga and detail all your hopes and   aspirations.
Task:
Why was Kundalini yoga kept a secret?
Task:
Explain   Hot   yoga
Task:
How   is   Iyengar   yoga   different?
Please note that these self-assessment

tasks are to ensure your understanding of the information within each module. As such, do not submit them for review with KEW Training Academy.

CHAPTER 4: WHAT IS YOGA?

"Yoga is an ancient art based on a harmonizing system of development for the body, mind, and spirit" (yoga,org). The earliest writings and teachings on yoga were actually written on palm leaves about 5,000 years ago. However, some researchers believe that yoga is around 10,000 years old.

So, what does all of this mean? What really is yoga?

Yoga was used first by an ancient civilization in India and was a "mishmash" of various ideas, techniques and purposes. Many people do yoga for stress relief, health, fitness and flexibility. However, there are many reasons to practice yoga. Yoga has so many benefits like improving health problems like asthma, obesity, irritable bowel syndrome and more. Yoga can also help with mental illnesses, as it calms the mind.

Yoga has also been used to treat people with ADHD (attention deficit hyperactivity disorder) to calm the mind and to allow the person to find focus.

People think that all yoga is about is enhancing or improving something on your own body. But really, it's about taking time out your busy life and listening to what your body is saying and knowing what you need to do to relax. For many people, yoga is a way of life or even a way of getting away from life.

The Benefits of Yoga

So, officially, what are the benefits of yoga?

As stated earlier, yoga can be used to enhance many parts of the body and can help with a variety of physical, mental or emotional problems.

Some of the physical benefits, we have already mentioned including increased flexibility, muscle strength, tone, and energy, quickened metabolism and also weight loss.

The poses in yoga often have a little stretch to them, helping with tight or sore muscles and can even make you more flexible. Some poses are designed just to enhance flexibility and stretch muscles.

There are also many poses in the practice that promote muscle building and tone. Some of the moves or poses in yoga are considered body weight exercises. This is linked to a method of exercise called calisthenics. Calisthenics is known for stress relief and extreme weight loss. This is how yoga can be used for weight loss and muscle building (to an extent). The combination of eating well and body weight yoga moves can help you lose weight efficiently. Making yoga and eating well a habit can also help you keep off the weight.

Weight loss and yoga are also connected in the way that yoga helps people be more mindful or what they are doing and of what they put into their bodies. When you are more mindful, you can even tell when you really are hungry, as well. This way over eating will not be so much of a problem as it was before. Knowing when to stop eating is also another benefit of being mindful.

If you have problems with your posture, yoga can help with that as well. Many poses require a straight back and square shoulders. Doing these poses daily, or even a few times a week can help you build the good habit of sitting and standing up straight; straight enough to balance a book on your head.

You'll notice that as your flexibility increases as you practice yoga, your joints will also feel a sense of freedom. This may be a long term effect of yoga. It is proven that yoga can "prevent cartilage and joint breakdown." This is due to the stretch and movement of joints in their full range of motion.

It is well known that body weight exercises promote healthy and stronger bones. Yoga is no different. We've already talked about how some poses are based on holding your own body weight and intern, this can promote healthier, stronger bones in time.

Yoga is said to also help with blood pressure problems. If you have high blood pressure and you take some time out of your day to relax, stretch and focus on your breathing, it is proven that you can improve your high blood pressure drastically.

Of course, there are mental benefits as well. This includes helping with stress—and then intern back and neck ache, sleeping problems, headaches and more. If you illuminate stress than many of the daily struggles you have mentally can be illuminated as well.

Other than stress, yoga can have a great impact on your mental clarity and overall mental wellness. This is due to the meditation-style of some yoga. Focusing on your breathing and taking time to relax and stretch out with some yoga can help you achieve calmness, relax your mind, relieve chronic stress, and improve concentration.

So why is yoga so good for reducing stress and mental health? Let's go back to high school biology class when you learned about the human nervous system.

We learned about something called the sympathetic and parasympathetic nervous systems. The sympathetic nervous system is what controls the "fight or flight" response that our body has when we are in times of stress. The parasympathetic nervous system is simply what controls the cool down after that time of stress. In simpler terms, we go from super stressed to calmer.

The reason why we are relearning some high school biology is due to the idea that yoga allows us to go from that fight or flight response all the way to the calmer place that we like to go and stay. When your day was really bad or when you are panicking for some reason, you can take five minutes to calm down with some yoga poses.

Another reason why yoga is just so good for mental health is due to the fact that it gives you a chance to have a conversation with yourself, or really understand what bothered you today. This gives you a chance to confront those feelings or thoughts, or to decide whether or not they are important enough to worry about.

Why is Yoga Important?

Yoga has been used by doctors to cure or improve many mental disorders. Some of these diseases or disorders include ADHD (attention deficit hyperactivity disorder), SAD (seasonal affective disorder), depression, and chronic stress and anxiety. Yoga is such a good treatment for many of these diseases due to its calming nature an - as mentioned previously - its many mental health benefits.

Yoga is also very important in many religions, including Hinduism, Jainism and Buddhism. However, it is important to realize that practicing yoga does not mean you are not practicing another religion other than your own; many people believe this at first. You do not have to worry, you will not be offending the higher power that you follow.

Yoga is simply a lifestyle or a way of living life. This is comparable to eating healthy and exercising. Leading a healthy lifestyle is just the way you live, and has little to nothing to do with your religious beliefs. Yoga has also been proven to promote self-healing.

Yoga is important for many different reasons; the ones that you've read here are just the beginning. You'll find that many yoga poses are designed solely for certain reasons. Within the next few chapters, you'll find many different poses that are designed for weight loss, mental clarity or mental issues and focus.

How Long to Hold Each Exercise

Generally speaking, the benchmark for holding each exercise is when you start breathing hard and holding the pose becomes physically uncomfortable. At that point, you should continue exercising for about fifteen more seconds before relaxing. The reason for exercising after the point of uncomfortably is because this how you improve your endurance.

Footwork and Balance

It might seem like the footwork is being oversimplified. It is. The reason for this is because you're fat and out of shape. The point of this book is to put you into a position to succeed. Success begins with proper footwork. Over time, you'll become more coordinated and more flexible. Stick to the guidelines until you can hold the pose without wobbling or falling.

Asana (The Prayer Pose)

Type: Isometric.

Develops: Upper body strength and endurance.

Position: Standing with feet normal width apart.

Alternate Position: Seated with feet on the floor normal width apart and back straight.

Description: Put your hands together, palms facing inward. The fingers and thumbs should be touching each other and your thumbs should be touching your chest. Your forearms should be parallel to the ground.

Exercise: Push your hands together as hard as you are able. Keep your head, neck, lower back and legs relaxed. Exert even pressure until you begin to feel discomfort in your arms or you begin to breathe hard. Maintain the exercise for about 15 seconds after you feel discomfort or notice that you are breathing hard.

Notes: This position is based upon a traditional Hindu greeting. Trekkers may also recognize this as a traditional Vulcan greeting.

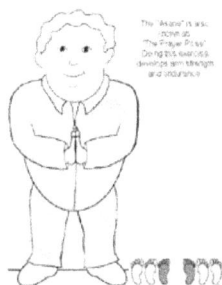

Atlas (The Beer Vendor Pose)

Type: Isometric.

Develops: Overall strength and endurance.

Position: Standing under a doorway with the front foot extended.

Alternate Position: **None.**

Description: Place the palms of your hands on the top of the doorframe. Extend your arms and lock your elbows. Keep your back straight; relax your head and neck. The feet are normal width apart. Extend one foot forward while keeping both heels firmly on the ground.

Exercise: Press vertically against the door frame with all your might. Keep your head and neck relaxed. Exert steady pressure until you begin to begin to breathe hard or feel discomfort in your arms, legs or back. Maintain the exercise for about 15 seconds after you notice that you are breathing hard or feeling discomfort in your arms legs or back.

Notes: This exercise is based on the mythical figure Atlas. You can also picture this exercise as a beer vendor carrying a case of beer through the bleachers at Wrigley Field.

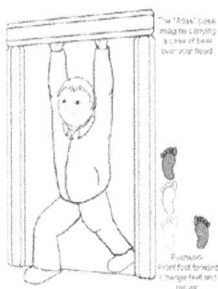

The Bridge

Type: Isometric.

Develops: Abdominal strength, leg strength and endurance.

Position: Lay flat on your back on a firm surface. Do not use your bed or a couch. The knees are bent and the soles of the feet rest flat on the ground. Your arms are relaxed at your sides and your head and neck are relaxed. You should use a mat if you have one.

Alternate Position: **None.**

Description: Your lower back, buttocks and legs are raised, forming a small arch.

Exercise: Flex your buttocks while slowly raising your pelvis off the floor. It should feel like the bones of your spine are coming up off the floor one after another. You should stop raising your pelvis when you feel your shoulder blade began to lift. If you raise your shoulder blades off the floor, you'll put too much stress on your neck. Maintain that position until you feel discomfort in your abdomen or legs or until you begin to breathe hard. Maintain the exercise for about 15 seconds after you notice the discomfort or that you are breathing hard.

If your legs cramp during this exercise, stop immediately.

Notes: This exercise is a variant of a wrestling drill known as "bridging".

You can help keep your upper spine properly aligned by placing a rolled up towel under your neck during this exercise.

If you cramp up during this exercise, walk it off and refer to the section on cramping at the end of the book.

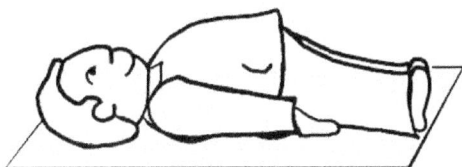

Bridge Resting Position:
needs no explanation...

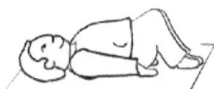

Bridge Start Position.
Feet normal width apart,
hands and heels on the floor

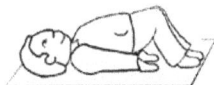

Bridge Exercise Position.
Flex your butts and slowly raise down off the floor
Remember: Do not lift your shoulderblades

The Plank

Type: Isometric.

Develops: Overall body strength and endurance.

Position: The up position of the push-up.

Alternate Position: **None.**

Description: The "up position" of the push-up (many of you may consider this position mythical or legendary).

Exercise: Hold the position until you begin to breathe hard or you experience discomfort in your arms, then hold the position for about 15 more seconds.

If your arms cramp up during this exercise, stop immediately.

Notes: This exercise can be made more challenging by placing the feet on an object so that the feet are above the hands.

Work hard to keep your spine properly aligned during this exercise.

If you cramp up during this exercise, walk it off and refer to the section on cramping at the end of the book.

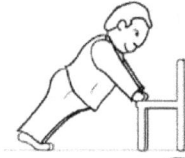

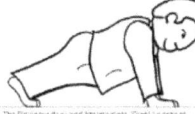

This Beginner (top) and Intermediate "Plank" positions.

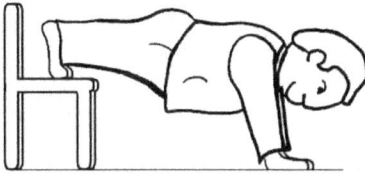

The Advanced "Plank" position with the feet above the hands.

The Power Position

Type: Isometric.

Develops: Lower body strength and endurance.

Position: Sit in a chair with your arms and hands extended over your head. Clench your fists and lock your elbows. Look straight ahead, relax your neck and keep your back straight.

Alternate Position: Clasp your hands together above your head.

Description: A modified sitting position.

Exercise: Lift your buttocks about three inches off of the chair. Hold this position until you begin breathing hard or began to feel discomfort in your legs. Then hold the position for 15 more seconds.

Stop the exercise and sit down immediately if your legs cramp up, you lose your balance or otherwise feel this position has become unsafe.

Notes: This exercise is also used for self evaluation purposes.

Work hard to keep your spine properly aligned during this exercise.

If you cramp up during this exercise, walk it off and refer to the section on cramping at the end of the book.

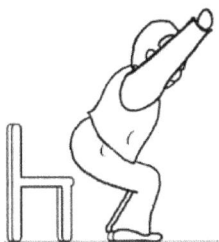

The "Power Plex" is used to determine if your baseline indicates if your baseline is at a steady rate for measuring improvement.

Samson

Type: Isometric.

Develops: Upper body strength and endurance.

Position: Stand in a doorway with your feet normal width apart.

Alternate Position: **None.**

Description: Stand in a doorway and extend your arms. Grasp the door frame at about shoulder height. Look straight ahead and relax your head and neck.

Exercise: Press outward with all of your might against the door frame until you feel discomfort in your arms or you begin to breathe hard. Then hold the pose for about 15 more seconds.

Notes: This pose is named after the biblical hero Samson.

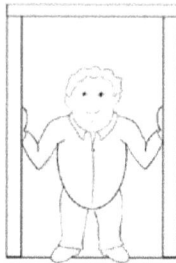

The 'Samson' position, keep your first normal width apart

Toe Lifts

Type: Isotonic.

Develops: Lower leg strength, endurance and balance.

Position: Stand with your knees locked and your feet normal width apart. Place your toes on the edge of a stair with your heels hanging over the edge. Keep your head and neck relaxed while looking straight ahead.

Alternate Position: You can use any elevated step. Many vehicles have excellent platforms for this exercise as well. Some examples include the tailgate of a golf cart, the side doors of most minivans and the running boards of many medium duty trucks.

Description: A modified standing position.

Exercise: Raise or lower your feet to a predetermined position and hold that position until you breathe hard. Then relax for 15 seconds and repeat three times.

Alternate Exercise: Raise and lower your body using only your toes. Move smoothly and evenly through your full range of motion several times until you get tired, then continue for about fifteen more seconds.

Notes: You can even do this exercise while waiting for the bus. Simply let your heels hang over the edge of the curb and use the bus stop sign for balance. If anybody asks what you are doing, you can tell them you are superhero preparing for a day of fighting villainy. It's (probably) not true, but it's fun to see how people react.

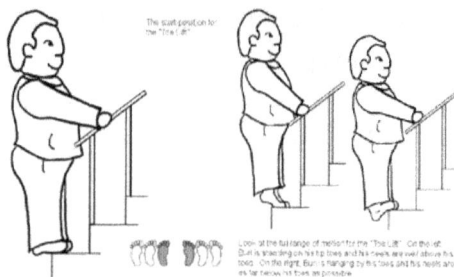

X Factor Arms (Wolverine)

Type: Isometric.

Develops: Upper body strength and endurance.

Position: Stand with your feet normal width apart. Look forward while relaxing your head and neck. Cross your arms in front of your chin with the forearms touching.

Alternate Position: You can do this exercise sitting down or laying on a mat.

Description: A modified standing position.

Exercise: Press your forearms together with all your might. Hold this position for about 15 seconds after you begin breathing hard. Relax for one minute, reverse the position of your arms and repeat.

Notes: Feel free to tape kitchen knives to your knuckles during this exercise. You will look and feel just like Wolverine ^{tm}.

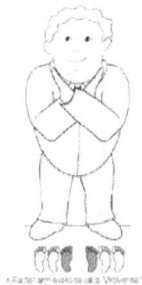

X Factor Legs

Type: Isometric.

Develops: Lower body strength and endurance.

Position: Lay down on a smooth, firm surface. Support your neck with a towel. Relax your head and neck and look upward. Rest your arms in any comfortable position. Bring your knees up to your chest and cross your lower legs above the ankle.

Alternate Position: **None.**

Description: See start position.

Exercise: Press your legs together with all your might. Hold this position for about 15 seconds after you begin breathing hard. Relax for one minute, reverse the position of your legs and repeat.

Notes: If possible, keep your entire upper body relaxed during this exercise.

CHAPTER 6: CORPSE POSE☐

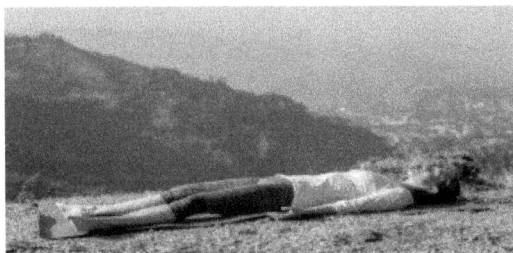

Also known as 'Savasana,' this gentle pose nevertheless forms an important part of a regular yoga practice. Your aim to get your body aligned in a 'neutral' position, which alleviates stress on your skeletal structure as well as your internal organs. Once you are in this pose, watch your breathing and embrace the opportunity to relax. Try beginning and ending your yoga practice with this asana. Begin by sitting on your yoga mat, feet flat on the floor with your knees bent. Lower your pelvis to the floor in one smooth motion. Inhale. As you do so, extend your right then left leg so that they are both in full contact with the floor beneath you. Your legs should be spread shoulder-width apart with your feet relaxed and turned out to the sides. Inhale again, then exhale as you lay back on the mat, back in straight alignment. Keep your head aligned - your ears should each be of a similar distance from your shoulders. Finally, stretch your arms straight up towards the ceiling, as though you are reaching for a distant object. Holding your arms still in this position, gently move your torso side to side. Feel your ribcage and shoulders flattening and spreading onto the mat. Lower your arms and hands, bringing them down flat against the mat so that your palms are facing the sky. Remain in this asana for 3-5 minutes. When it is time to finish your practice, exhale and roll up onto one side. Breathe a few more times, and then with a final exhalation push your hands to the mat an d bring your body upright to a seated position. The head should always come up last.

Bound Angle Pose☐

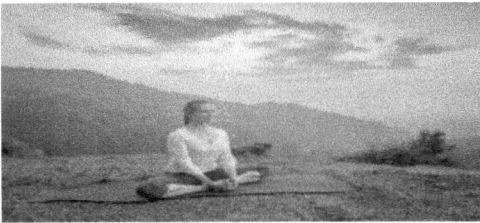

This pose, also known as 'Baddhakonasana' is excellent for improving your hip flexibility and general posture. To begin with, sit on your mat. Keep your back upright, and stretch your legs out in front of you. Take a couple of deep breaths. As you exhale, bring your heels together as you bend your knees. Draw your feet towards your pelvis, keeping the soles in full contact as you lower your knees to the floor. As you do this, you should feel a gentle stretch in your thighs and groin.

Aim to keep the outer edges of your feet flat to the floor as you hold onto the big toe of each foot. Your pelvis should be in a neutral position, with your perineum in line with the floor. Sit up as straight as you can. Do not round your shoulders. If you find it hard to draw your knees down to the floor, instead imagine that you are lowering your thigh bones. This change of prospective can help some new practitioners find their way into this asana.

If you find this pose difficult, sitting on a folded blanket or block can help you move into position. Remember to take it slowly - yoga is not a race! - and do what you can. If you commit to practicing regularly, you will find that your flexibility increases naturally and that in time you will no longer have to use such props.

Remain in Bound Angle Pose for 1-5 minutes, depending on your comfort level. Yoga should never hurt or cause you notable discomfort, so if you start to feel any significant and unpleasant sensations, exit the position. To do this, take a deep breath. As you inhale, imagine drawing your thighs back upwards to their original position.

Tree Pose☐

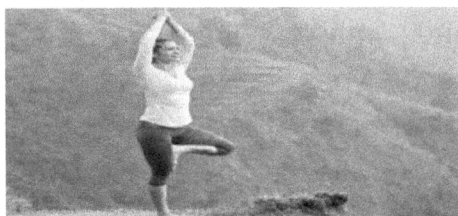

Also known as 'Vrikshasana,' the Tree Pose is an excellent way of developing good posture, increasing your balance, and developing core strength.

Begin by standing with your feet together. Take a few deep breaths, imagining a cord running through your spine and through the top of your head. Picture this cord as taut, pulling your chin upwards so that your neck and spine are in natural alignment. Let your arms hang loosely on each side of your body.

Inhale, and pull your right foot upwards so that the sole of your foot is flat against your left inner thigh. Place the heel of your foot as high up on your thigh as possible. Now comes the most difficult part - finding your sense of balance! Draw your abdominal muscles back towards your spine, keep your head and neck aligned, and look straight ahead. Place your hands above your head, palms together and elbows bent in a prayer-like position. Keep your left leg straight. Pressing your right heel more firmly into your thigh can help retain a sense of balance.

It is usual practice in other yoga asanas to close one's eyes, which can help keep your focus on your breath. However, Tree Pose is much easier if you keep your eyes open!

Hold this pose for 2-5 minutes. The first few times you attempt this asana, 30 seconds may feel like an achievement. Don't worry if finding your balance proves difficult. Simply keep practicing and congratulate yourself for taking the first steps on your path to a regular yoga practice.

Cobra Pose☐

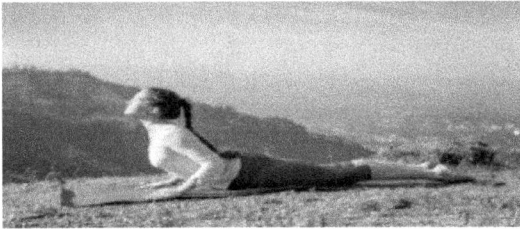

Cobra Pose ('Bhujangasana') is an excellent pose for opening up the chest and strengthening the shoulders.

Start by lying face-down on the mat. Extend your legs as far as they will comfortably go. The tops of your feet should be in contact with the mat. Place your hands, palms-down, on the floor directly underneath your shoulders. Your elbows should be in close contact with the sides of your body. Take a deep breath. As you exhale, press your feet, thighs and pelvis to the floor.

Inhale, and as you do so straighten your arms in such a way that your chest comes away from the mat. Keep straightening your arms until you can no longer keep your pelvis, thighs and feet aligned and in contact with the floor. Resist the urge to harden your buttocks. They should be held firm, but not clenched. Open your shoulders, and ensure that your spine is evenly bent all the way down. Keep your breathing regular as you remain in this position for 30 seconds. Exhale as you smoothly lower your body back to the ground.

Yoga though most people associate it with religion, is actually not affiliated to religion per se but is the earliest form of physical discipline recorded in human life on earth. It is an ancient kind of exercise that greatly focuses on flexibility, strength, and breathing in order to not only boost your physical well being but also mental well being.

The exact origin of yoga is debatable. However, it is thought to be around fifty centuries old. The earliest known sighting of yoga according to experts traces back to around 3000 B.C. The word 'yoga' is derived from Sanskrit and translates to merge or unite. Yoga is a form of exercise of the body and mind, which is based upon the intimate connection between the body, breathing, and mind. By manipulation of breathe and stabilizing the body in poses, yoga achieves harmony. Through yoga, you can balance and regulate your body, mind, and in-depth feelings to withdraw themselves from the chaos of the world and find inner peace. Yoga achieves this by using movement, breathe, stability, relaxation and meditation to construct a healthy, stable and a positive approach to life.

Yoga, as seen through the eyes of modern scientists, is defined as a science that helps an individual search for their soul and establishes unity between the individual of finite existence and the infinite divine spiritual force. Control and balance are what you could really benefit while practicing yoga, apart from other advantages. In every aspect of life, yoga represents balanced moderation. Since yoga has evolved over time, let us have a closer look at modern yoga

Modern Yoga

The system of yoga followed now in most western countries is called Hatha yoga. The word 'Hatha' derived from Sanskrit is a composite of Ha, which means 'sun' and

Tha, which means 'moon'. Hatha Yoga is the union between two separate entities, interdependent but separate. This is suggestive of the healthy collaboration of extremes - in this case, the mind and body, which leads to strength, vitality and a feeling of satisfaction.

Hatha yoga is strongly based on the practice of postures (called asanas), various breathing techniques (called pranayama) and meditation (called Dhyana) for overall development. It aims to regulate the flow of energy in and out of the body as a form of exercise. The asanas or postures emphasize on controlled movement, focus, flexibility, and deep breathing. There are nearly 200 asanas of which more than half are practiced widely in the world. The postures vary from very simple to complex. Even though, the movements are slower and controlled, Hatha Yoga provides you with a complete and thorough workout for the mind and body. Before we can go on to choosing suitable asanas, it is important that you understand yoga is not a religion. Although yoga is associated with spirituality, it is not the ideal definition of a religion. Hatha yoga is a physical and psychological discipline that integrates the learning and practice of asanas, pranayama, and meditation.

While yoga is purely not a religion, there are certain spiritual ethics associated with it in the practice. These yoga principles include five yamas, which follow paths of non-violence, truthfulness, honesty, chastity, and generosity. There is another set of five principles called niyamas, which symbolize purity, contentment, self-discipline, self-study, and divine spirituality.

Now that you have some basic understanding of yoga, let us now look at yoga poses for weight loss in the following chapter.

CHAPTER 8: FLEXIBILITY AND STRENGTH OF THE BODY

Enhanced flexibility is among the most important advantages of yoga. If you are brand new to yoga, you may not even be capable of touching your feet without help.

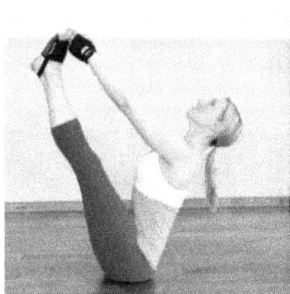

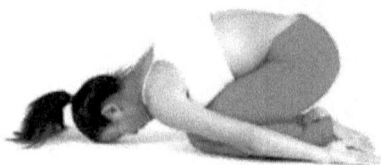

But if you continue to practice, you will notice a steady increase in flexibility which reduces the risk of injury and lessens the duration of symptoms associated with injury.

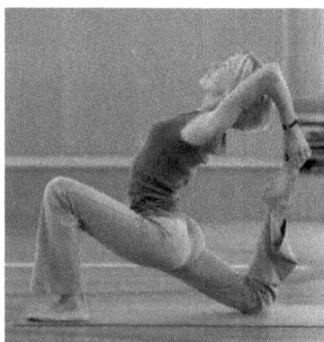

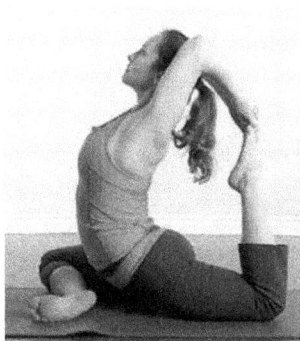

Strong muscles are for more than just looking great. They guard against inflammation of the joints, lessen the injury threshold associated with falls in elderly people and prevent lower, middle and upper back pain.

UPWARD DOG

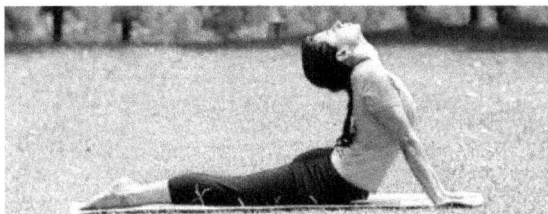

TO CURE OBESITY

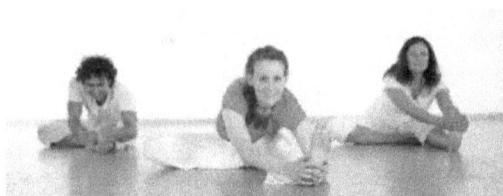

Part of connecting the mind and body is the ability to start to eat intuitively. One of the benefits of a regular yoga practice is experiencing a regulation of the appetite.

In addition, the body may very well start to crave healthy foods and acknowledge how it is affected by eating food that is not healthy.
Standing Positions

Our mind is similar to a game ball— big, spherical, and large. If it is nicely placed straight above erect spine, it takes a smaller amount work with the spinal muscles to aid it.

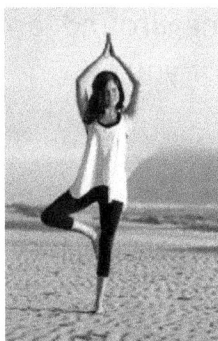

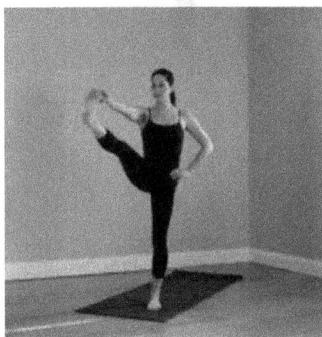

Without proper alignment of the head and neck your head you will begin to experience bad posture and possibly straining your neck muscles.

That muscle strain can have a direct effect on energy levels. If you're energy is going toward holding up your head in an uncomfortable position while sitting at a desk or walking around on the job, less energy is left for you.

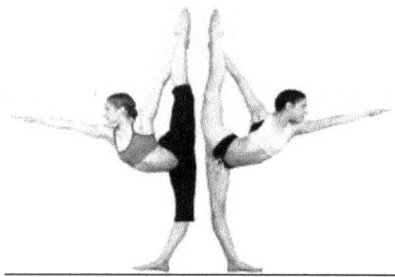

Bad posture may cause back pain, neck pain and joint pain. If you continually practice bad posture, your body will compensate and unnecessary strain will be placed on other joints and muscles.

Vertebrae disks—the absorbers involving the spinal backbone that will herniate and shrink nerves— crave motion.

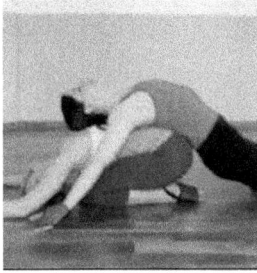

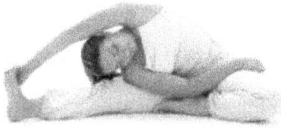

BACK PAIN RELIEF SIDE BEND

If you've got a well-balanced practice with plenty of   backbends, forward bends, and strong standing and floor postures, yoga postures, you will keep your spine strong, healthy and elastic.

A strong and healthy spine can prevent degenerative   arthritis   in the backbone.

Asthma

Research indicates that engaging in a regular yoga practice can reduce asthma and allergy symptoms and minimize the need for medication to treat the ailments.

This does not mean you should avoid medicinal treatments when experiencing a bronchial asthma attack. It simply suggests that a regular yoga practice could alleviate the symptoms and lessen the severity of attacks.

ASTHMA RELIEF POSE

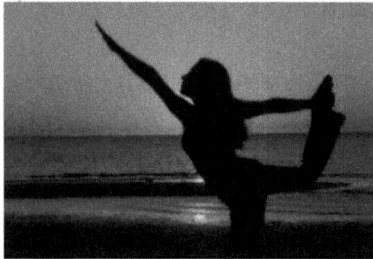

Research suggests
that this practice regulates our physical and emotional stress responses and our coping mechanisms. Meditation and yoga have long since been used to treat

depression and stress related conditions.A consistent yoga practice provides physical movement, burns energy, and allows us to connect with ourselves mentally and spiritually on a deeper level.

The most important pieces of yoga, the breathing exercises, have been known to enhance lung performance. The ability to "catch one's breath" and breathe steadily is said to be the true measure of physical fitness.

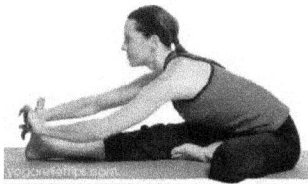

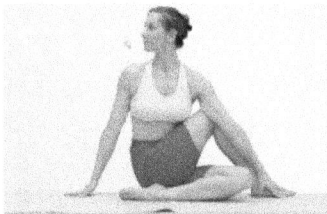

FOR DIGESTION FLEXIBLE NECK

Yoga   promotes breathing slowly   and deeply   through   the nose.   Pranayama breathing, using 100 % of the lung power, is believed to detox the lungs and exercise them   making   them   stronger   and   more resilient. Rapid   breathing   through   the mouth sends us into panic mode and does not   allow   our   heart   rate   to   regulate.

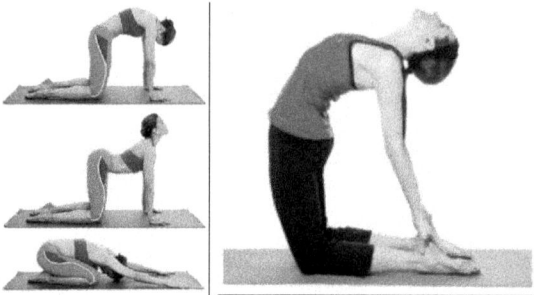

CAT   COW   STRETCHCAMEL   FOR CONCENTRATION

An essential element of yoga is actually emphasizing the existing situation. Numerous reports have found that regular yoga practice increases co-ordination, reaction time, memory, and one's ability to reason.

Yoga encourages you to relax, concentrate on the breath and focus on the current, moving the balance in the sympathetic nervous system towards the parasympathetic nervous system.

The latter is relaxing as well as regenerative; this decreases inhaling and exhaling as well as cardiovascular rates, decreases blood pressure, and increases blood flow to the intestines and the reproductive system organs.

Improve Self Respect

Most of us have problems with persistently reduced self-pride. Should you choose to handle this negatively—

take medications, eat   way   too   much,
function too   hard, sleep around—
you might pay the   price   as   a less   wholly
healthy   person
bodily, emotionally, and spiritually.

If you take a confident approach and practice yoga, your perception will shift, first in brief glimpses but then more continually until you realize you are worthwhile and that you are the representative of the Divine.

When you practice yoga regularly with the goal of self-contemplation and betterment,
you can access a different part of yourself you may not otherwise have known existed.

You'll experience emotions related of gratitude, concern for others and a feeling that you are a part of something bigger.

People who train in Transcendental Yoga demonstrate the ability to master difficulties and obtain and recall information better— probably as they are less distracted by their feelings.

FOR JOINTS

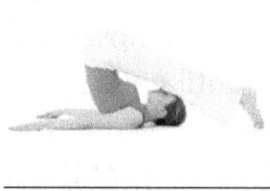

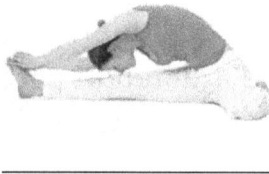

Do   you   ever notice yourself tightly
gripping a steering   wheel,
perhaps scrunching the face while looking
at a computer screen, or even holding
your breath for no reason?

These unconscious habits can   result
in persistent anxiety,   muscle
mass fatigue, and   pain in
the wrists, biceps,   triceps,   shoulder
blades, neck   which   can increase your
stress levels   and
aggravate your disposition.

Yoga can help you to be conscious of these movements and fix them so they do not manifest in to physical issues.

FOR HIP JOINTS

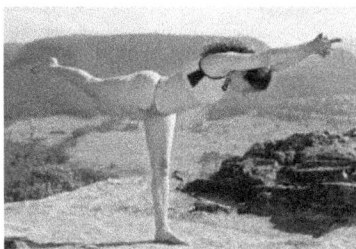

When you practice, you begin to notice places you hold stress and anxiety; it may be in your tongue, your eyes, or perhaps the muscles of the face and neck or in the clenching of your jaw. By simply tuning in to your body, you can address these subconscious behaviors and practice relaxation.

KNEE JOINTELBOW JOINT

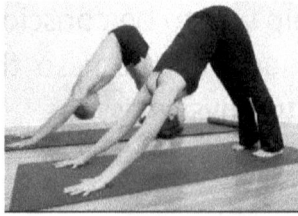

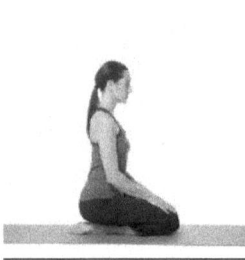

With bigger muscle groups such as the quadriceps, hamstrings and hips, it might take numerous practices until you start to notice these muscle groups loosening up.

Yoga, like any exercise, can ease constipation—and the theory is that reduction of constipation reduces the risk of intestinal tract cancer—because moving your body facilitates moving waste material more rapidly through the bowels.

FOR STOMACH

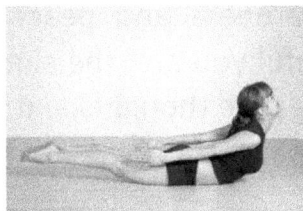

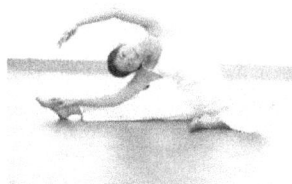

Yoga quenches the   actual imbalances of
the brain, based   on   **Patanjali's** Yoga
Sanskrit   literature. Quite
simply, this decreases the emotional loops
of disappointment, regret, frustration, fear
and desire that can cause stress.

Because anxiety is actually suggested as a
factor in so   many health problems—
from migraine   headaches to   insomnia,
hypertension   to   auto-immune   diseases,

reducing anxiety with yoga can be useful in managing anxiety which trickles down in relieving its side effects.

Yoga as well as meditation helps us to develop awareness and peacefulness. The more peaceful you are, the simpler it is to let go of negative thoughts and feelings.

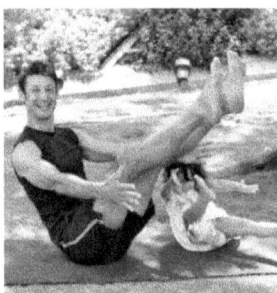

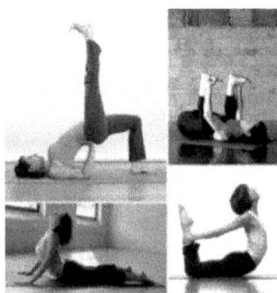

Before you begin, there are just some important things that you must keep in mind. Read on the following before signing up in a yoga class:

Know your body's capabilities—it is important that you do not force your body into a position that you find complicated, or at least beyond your body's limit. Yoga is not a sport, it is a form of exercise that helps release tension and pressures brought by everyday activities.

Bring yourself gently into apose—and when you hold a pose, listen to what your body tells you. Are there tensions building up? Should you feel anything unfamiliar, immediately relax that specific body part where you feel the tension from, loosen up, and breathe. Your progress may be slow, but with time, your body will get use to the positions.

Do not forget to check with your doctor first–yoga can be practiced by just about anyone–children, pregnant women, old people and the like. While there is no one to exclude, it is still important that you check with your doctor before starting a course, especially if you have a medical condition.

Proper Diet–there is a recommended diet for a yogi. It should be a simple vegetarian diet made up of all-natural food that are easy to digest. Why these? Aside from being heathy, they also calm the mind and free it from restless thoughts as compared to what processed food provide.

What you will need–to practice yoga, you need not have special gym equipment. All you need is a yoga mat or even a towel will do. If you are practicing indoors, it is ideal to go to a place with less furniture. The room should also have proper ventilation and free from any kind of disturbances.

A qualified yoga instructor is recommended–whether you are with a group or by yourself, it is advisable that you do it under the supervision of a trained and qualified instructor. A teacher will help with each pose and demonstrate proper ways to ease the body with different yoga poses. This is also to ensure that you do not put too much pressure on a particular body part.

The best time to practice yoga–It is recommend that you do it every day. But remember not to force yourself. Yoga must be an enjoyable and relaxing form of exercise. So pick a specific time of the day when no one will disturb you and you will not have to hurry with each position because of an errand. You can practice in the morning to help relieve tensed muscles from sleep. Or, you can do it in the evening to loosen muscles and tensions of the day.

For how long will each session last?–90 minutes is the recommend time. But you can also do it at shorter sessions. What is important is you do not rush each pose and make time for relaxation in between poses.

Chapter 10: What Yoga Is And Isn't

Yoga is far more than just a series of stretching exercises.It's not some kind or religion or cult, and it doesn't require one to turn into a vegan or sell all of their worldly possessions!It's nothing like its stereotype. Yoga first came to the Western hemisphere in 1893 at the World's Fair in Chicago.It was brought by Swami Vivekananda who was one of India's most popular gurus. The word yoga gets its origins from the Sanskrit word "Yug".It means to bind or join.Basically it is about unity of the physical body with the mind.It's about "conscious living".It's not all about calisthenics.

While the physical aspects are certainly an important part, this is not the only true purpose.It's also about the mental benefits. It's not any type of religion.There are no gods to worship, and it is not an organized system at all.Any spiritual benefits are purely emotional and psychological. Yoga doesn't actually distinguish between the physical body and the mind.Yoga can work to improve your physical health in many ways, not just aiding in weight loss, but also improving tone and even reducing physical pain.

Yoga allows you to release the tension that can build up in your body.It helps the various parts of your body become lose and limber, from your muscles and joints to your tendons and ligaments. It can help back pain, joint pain, muscle pain, and much more.People aren't meant to be stiff and rigid.We were designed to be flexible creatures.We may not all have the flexibility and grace of a prima ballerina, but we should all be healthy and fit.Yoga is one means to achieving such a goal. Here are some of the benefits that have been proven to exist through yoga:

Improved flexibility

Better range of motion

More fluid motion

Immune system strengthening

Reduced joint pain

Reduced muscular pain

Better breathing

Higher lung capacity

Higher metabolism

Better sleep quality

Reduced stress and anxiety

There are many other remarkable benefits reported to be received from yoga.You may discover many more. Yoga is beneficial in many ways.It's not all about the physical effects, as I've mentioned previously.Yoga may have its roots in the spiritual, but its foundation is based in science.Yoga's health benefits have been proven time and time again by many sources.Its physical benefits can be paramount to a healthy lifestyle.But of course there are mental and emotional benefits, as well.Yoga helps you achieve a type of mind/body harmony through the use of:

Postures (called asana)Breathing (called pranayama)Meditation (which we will cover later)All three of these are essential for obtaining the full benefit of yoga.For example, you may believe your breathing has nothing to do with your physical shape, but that's not true.Your body needs oxygen to function properly, and the more efficient your respiration is, the better your body can perform. Likewise meditation can also help you physically.When you meditate you relieve muscle tension.This can ease all kinds of aches and pains including back pain, joint pain, and even stress and anxiety.

There are a number of direct physical benefits that can be obtained from yoga when you use the three principles together:

Central nervous system harmony

Decrease in heart rate

Lower blood pressure

Better efficiency of your cardiovascular system

Gastrointestinal system improvement

Improved flexibility and dexterity

Better balance

Better memory and mental clarity

Depth perception improvement

There are a number of psychological benefits, too:

Can help break a smoking habit

Can help curb binge drinking

Can help you eat healthier

Can help ease insomnia

Can reduce stress and anxiety

Can decrease panic attacks

Can ease depression

Can help lethargy

While yoga isn't a cure-all and results won't happen overnight, it can certainly help you make some big changes to your psychological and physiological states. There are even some claims out there that yoga can ease the symptoms of many other illnesses, like diabetes.This has never been proven by medical science, but some people claim it can reduce the need for insulin by up to 50%.Yoga is also something that is relatively easy on the body.You can tailor a yoga workout to your own fitness level, and increase the difficulty as you progress.There's no reason you shouldn't be able to perform at least some of the asana no matter what physical condition you're in.As long as you have some mobility in your arms and legs, you should be able to start out with some of the easier asana and gradually increase the intensity of your yoga workout as you progress.

Don't overdo it.Too much of a good thing can be bad for you.You want to use yoga to improve your physical condition, not make it worse.If you overdo it, you may end up injuring yourself.This could make existing conditions worse and also set back any progress you've made so far. At the very least an injury could cause you to miss several days of workouts, which could hamper your progress, so it's best to take it easy until you get used to it.

CHAPTER 11: YOGA FOR BEGINNERS

Back bending, headstands, chanting, twisting to the left and right and up and down -- these images may pop up in your head when you think about yoga. Or you might think that it's this Indian fad with people on yoga mats and doing cartwheels.

Yes, you will perhaps need to stand on one leg and keep your feet over your leg but this is not just what yoga is all about. Yoga is a spiritual practice that dates back thousands and thousands of years ago. You may have noticed the multiple yoga studies appearing in your neighborhood or the increase in number of people you know that are recommending yoga. Some of it might tell you they're doing it to lose weight, some others to relax, while some are just there to try out this craze. But the bottom line is: **yoga is now one of the avenues entertained by people seeking a solution to their various problems.**

Long ago, the practice of yoga took a different form compared to the kind of yoga we are familiar with right now which is largely comprised of the asanas -- the postures -- that we practice. Nevertheless, one thing that hasn't changed is the objective of yoga. **Yoga** means union and as its name suggests, it aims to reunite the mind and the body.

There are many places that offer yoga teachings. You can go to yoga studios, gyms, and wellness centers where instructors are available to guide you through the whole process. However, it's no longer necessary to join a class and spend dollars on daily or weekly sessions since yoga is as easily done in your own home or even at work. Yoga can provide a lot of advantages to a person and this is pretty much a very big factor why so many people are making yoga their new hobby. Not only does it offer physical benefits but it can also improve one's mental wellbeing and help a person achieve inner peace and enlightenment.

Regarding its physical gains, it includes weight reduction, improved respiration, and better athletic performance. To add, practicing yoga will improve flexibility through the asanas that will require the stretching of body parts. As we age, it is normal to lose flexibility and experience pain and immobility when we try to move parts of our body. However, yoga can address this problem. You will be amazed by how your body can move and twist in ways you never expected it could.

Power poses like headstands demand you to support the weight of your own body. Practicing these poses for some time would build your strength. Additionally, as you get stronger, you can also expect toned muscles and a leaner body.

Furthermore, due to poses that require you to stand on one leg or invert yourself, balance can be improved.

Vis-à-vis the physical gains are the mental benefits that yoga can offer. It will teach you to calm your mind through the physical asanas that you have to perform. While you are doing your session, there will be no room for all your worries, doubts, and anxieties and you will learn to steer your thoughts away from what is unnecessary.

Yoga will also introduce you to meditation techniques that will aid you to become more mindful and achieve emotional tranquility and stability.

Moreover, one of the most important contributions of yoga is how it can reduce one's stress level. Since you will be mainly concentrating on the asanas and on your breathing, you won't have the luxury of beating yourself up and letting all those negative thoughts run around. While you are on the mat, any trouble you have in mind will not come to the fore.

Yoga will also provide you a better understanding of your body and make you appreciate what its capabilities are and how it can break through its limits. You will realize that your body and mind are both powerful and note-worthy. Beginners claim at first of not being able to perform the ideal forms of the asanas because of body complications but later on, they are amazed to find out that through practice and will power, they are able to twist their bodies in ways they never imaged was possible.

Yoga has different major branches and every branch of yoga focuses on certain types of objective and practice. It is advisable for beginners to be aware of the different types of yoga and find what kind is suitable for their personality and what can serve their purpose.

Raja Yoga

This branch of yoga puts a lot of emphasis on meditation. People who are interested and prefer exercises that require introspection usually engage in Raja yoga. Religious individuals and members of spiritual communities, for one, are into this type of yoga. Additionally, Raja yoga encourages its yogis to follow a monastic or contemplative kind of lifestyle.

Karma Yoga

Karma relates to action and to "doing". We relate the word **karma** to the idea that any action that we do has a consequence. This is the principle of karma yoga -- the experiences we are going through today are results of the past actions we committed and enacted. The main goal, therefore, of Karma yoga is to teach people to lead a life filled with causes that would generate more favorable and successful effects in the future.

Bhakti Yoga

For those whose primary goal in yoga is the attainment of wellbeing and emotional fulfillment, bhakti or devotional yoga is usually the preferred path. The **bhakta** often practices meditation, visualizing in the process that God is standing before him. One channels out the feelings from the heart and deepest thoughts with his or her God. Bhakti yoga is also considered the yoga of the heart.

Jnana Yoga

If bhakti yoga is the yoga of the heart, jnana yoga is considered as the yoga of the mind. Development of the intellect and procurement of knowledge through studying the scriptures related to the yogic tradition is one of the demands of this branch of yoga. The main goal of jnana meditation is to achieve transformation and enlightenment from all the thoughts and feelings that may prove detrimental and distracting to the soul and body.

Tantra Yoga

Unlike most people's understanding, tantra yoga is not about crude sexual practices for men and women. The pathway of rituals, it is concerned with a force that we can transform into higher channels and involves embracing a ritualistic approach towards life. The goal of this branch of yoga is the awakening and harmonization of the female and male facets of a human person. If you're the kind of person who's deeply interested and believed in the observance of rituals and ceremonies, tantra yoga might just be your kind of yoga.

Mantra Yoga

Mantras refer to chanted syllables, words, or phrases. In mantra yoga, meditating involves the chanting of a word or phrase until the chanting overcomes the mind and emotions and a new state of awareness is revealed.

Hatha Yoga

Hatha yoga provides a gentle introduction to yoga for beginners. Nowadays, it is mainly practiced for its health benefits because it targets both the mind and body during the exercises required in the sessions. It is mainly interested in the practice of asanas and how doing the poses would achieve a clearer mind and healthier body.

Kundalini Yoga

A combination of raja, tantra, hatha, laya, and matra yoga, kundalini is a method to reach a better state of self and achieve spiritual enlightenment. Doing kundalini yoga stimulates the main life energy coiled at the base of spine in order for this force to travel to the other spiritual centers in the body. The ultimate aim would be for the life force to reach the spiritual center at the crown of your head so you can experience a higher consciousness.

Kriya Yoga

Kriya yoga is a combination of jnana, bhakti, and raja yoga. The word **kriya** means "to transform." It aims to discipline the mind and body and encourage introspection. It also involves making the life force inside the body to move up and down one's spine in order to transform the yogi.

Once you've finally decided on the perfect branch of yoga that you want to delve into, it's finally time to get the ball rolling. You're ready for your first yoga session. However, there are some reminders that you must take into consideration.

What to eat

It is greatly encouraged not to eat 2 to 3 hours before practicing yoga. Since some of the asanas would demand physical contortions of the body, discomfort might be felt in the process if you haven't digested your last meal fully. However, for people with a fast metabolism, refraining from eating might lead to hunger and weakness during the session so you might as well partake in some light snack about an hour before the session.

What to bring

All you need to prepare is your towel, water bottle, and yoga mat. In yoga studios, they usually provide yoga mats but if you want to ensure that your yoga mat is clean and comfortable, you could buy one for your own. When you're at home or at work, it'd be encouraged to have your yoga mat around so your body has a sort of insulation against the cold, hard floor.

What to wear

Comfort is the key. During yoga sessions, wear clothes that you feel you're most comfortable with. People usually don on yoga pants and tank tops since they don't restrict one's movements. Tight jeans must be avoided for they won't allow proper execution of the ideal forms of the asanas.

Moreover, if you can afford not to, don't wear your eyeglasses during the session. Especially when you're doing the power postures, there is a great risk of damage to your spectacles when you're wearing them during asanas.

What to expect

Don't expect to immediately be able to execute all the asanas. If you're a beginner, you may not be able to do all the power poses yet especially the power poses that need a lot of flexibility and balance. But don't worry. With practice and time, you'll definitely be able to advance through the asanas.

Where, when, and how many times to practice

For people who refuse to spend bucks paying for an instructor in a formal yoga studio and decide on doing yoga sessions on their own, there will be no problem when it comes to practice space. All you need to find is a place with a flat surface where you'll be comfortable in. A space in your bedroom or living room will serve the purpose. You can then put your yoga mat on the floor to provide some cushion for your body.

As for the finest time to practice yoga, it should be during the early morning before breakfast. At this point in time, both body and mind have rested and fatigue-free. The favorable state in the morning will go a long way in boosting your determination to follow through your yoga sequence.

If you're not available during the early morning, you can choose to practice around sunset or early evening instead.

Obviously, daily practice is advisable in order to maximize the potential yoga can give you. But remember not to over-exert yourself. Don't spend 10 hours a day on yoga and perhaps just allot 2 hours for one yoga sequence.

Additionally, don't practice yoga when you're sick or in some kind of terrible pain. There are certain postures that you must avoid depending on you medical circumstances. Having high blood pressure, menstruation, injuries, and being pregnant would definitely affect your choice asanas.

You must always listen to your body and ignoring any warning of, "Hey, Joe. You might not want to practice today because my pancreas is dying" will never be encouraged. When you're sick, the physical exercises could worsen your situation. If you're unsure about the state of your body, consult your doctor first before you resume your sessions.

What to observe during session.

Any instruction manual or any yoga instructor would preach you the ideal form of the postures. Keyword is ideal. They are the goal but it doesn't necessarily mean that you have to break your back in order to do them. Modify the poses if necessary as long as the general legwork is still there.

In addition, it may not be advisable to talk during asanas as it would be a form of distraction especially if you're with other people.

Moreover, do not drink or eat during the practice proper. You should also choose and prepare your yoga sequence beforehand. Before you start your yoga program, mull over what postures you can do given your current level and remember the sequence of your postures. Don't stop midway through your yoga program just to leaf over your notes because you forgot what posture you intended to do next.

Chapter 12: Origin Of Yoga

Nobody knows precisely when Yoga started, however it absolutely originates before recorded history. Yoga positions portrayed by stone carving have been obtain in archeological destinations in the Indus Valley going back 5,000 years or more. There is a typical misguided judgment that Yoga is established in Hinduism; unexpectedly, Hinduism's religious structures developed much later and fused a portion of the acts of Yoga. (Different religions all through the world have likewise joined practices and thoughts identified with Yoga.)

The convention of Yoga has dependably been passed on independently from educator to understudy through oral instructing and reasonable exhibition. The formal strategies that are currently known as Yoga seem to be, hence, in light of the aggregate encounters of numerous people over numerous of great years. The specific way in which the systems are educated and rehearsed today relies upon the methodology went down in the line of educators supporting the individual expert.

One of the soonest messages doing with Yoga was gathered by a researcher named Patanjali, who set down the most predominant Yoga speculations and practices of his time in a book he called Yoga Sutras ("Yoga Aphorisms") as ahead of schedule as the first or second century B.C. then again as late as the fifth century A.D. (Unknown exact dates). The framework that he expounded on is known as "Ashtanga Yoga," or the eight limbs of Yoga, and this is what is for the most part alluded to today as Classical Yoga. Most present followers rehearse some variety of Patanjali's framework.

The eight stages of Classical Yoga are:

☐ Yama, signifying "limitation" — abstaining from viciousness, lying, taking, easygoing sex, and storing;

☐ Niyama, signifying "recognition" — virtue, happiness, resilience, study, and recognition;

☐Asana, physical activities;

☐Pranayama, breathing methods;

☐ Pratyahara, readiness for reflection, portrayed as "withdrawal of the brain from the faculties";

☐Dharana, fixation, having the capacity to hold the psyche on one item for a predetermined time;

☐Dhyana, contemplation, the capacity to concentrate on one thing (or nothing) inconclusively;

☐Samadhi, ingestion, or acknowledgment of the vital way of the self.

Modern Western Yoga classes widely concentrate on the third, fourth, and fifth steps. Yoga most likely touched base in the United States in the late 1800s, yet it didn't turn out to be broadly known until the 1960s, as a feature of the young society's developing enthusiasm for anything Eastern. As more got to be thought about the advantageous impacts of Yoga, it picked up acknowledgment and admiration as a profitable strategy for aiding in the administration of anxiety and enhancing wellbeing and prosperity. Numerous doctors now prescribe Yoga practice to patients at danger for coronary illness, and also those with back torment, joint inflammation, melancholy, and other interminable conditions.

WHAT IS YOGA?

Many of us have practiced Yoga for years, yet if someone asks us about a definition of what Yoga is, we would be hard pressed to give an answer. As many other important products of ancient Indian culture, Yoga isn't clearly defined and systematised like the scientific disciplines of the West. I will try to give a personal contribution to this subject; it is not a clear, simple definition I'm looking for, but rather an unveiling of the essence of this amazing science.

Modern definitions of Yoga.

Even though there aren't, in modern times, such famous definition as Patañjali's, it's still possible to identify some general approaches to Yoga.

Yoga as Fitness.

The main focus is placed on the practice of asanas (postures), and on the perfection of alignment. The therapeutic effects of each posture are sometimes studied in depth, so that a personalised practice can be devised, in order to address specific health conditions. In other styles of Yoga, the emphasis is on a powerful, dynamic practice that acts more as a prevention than a cure: which constantly stimulating energetic system and attaining a state of permanent physical balance and health.

Yoga as Meditation.

Another modern interpretation sees Yoga as primarily a meditation technique. Here, the focus is on calming and stabilising the mind, through the use of asanas, pranayama (breath control), as well as mental concentration techniques. This interpretation usually do not give so much importance to alignment in the postures, or to the physical benefits of Yoga; instead, the body is used as a tool to access one own's mind and gain more control over it.

Yoga as Union.

Some practitioners and schools understand Yoga as a process of union between one's own internal world (sometimes called the "Microcosm") and the Universe (the "Macrocosm"), Nature, or God. This interpretation are very focused on Bhakti (devotional) practices, such as Mantra chanting, rituals, and so on. The practice of postures, breathing exercises, and other techniques is seen as a tool to facilitate the union, or dissolution, of the individual Self into a higher, superior entity. The positive consequences on health, as well as the mental concentration that can be attained through the practice of Yoga, are seen as secondary effects, although beneficial.

Yoga as Evolution.

Yoga is a practical philosophical system whose objective is the physical, mental and spiritual evolution of the human being.

YOGA HELPS REDUCE STRESS

☐Yoga uses slow and deep belly breaths to lower your body's levels of the stress hormone cortisol.

☐ Yoga encourages people to practice "mindfulness," which can help combat stress over the long-term.

☐Non-impact moves help get the stress-relieving benefits of physical exercise.

When you're stressed to the max, climbing onto the yoga mat might not be your first move. But for some, it could be a smart one. Stress can contribute to headaches, and taking steps to reduce stress may help some people avoid them.

It Deepens Your Breathing

There's a reason people say, "take a deep breath." Deep breathing literally slows your sympathetic nervous system, which acts a lot like a gas pedal for your body. Yoga uses slow and most importantly, deep belly breaths to lower your body's levels of the stress hormone cortisol as well as supply your brain with more of the oxygen it needs to work at its best. The result: You're calmer and better able to solve the problems causing you stress.

It Teaches Mindfulness

When people are stressed, it could be because they're dwelling on the past or worrying about the future. Yoga, however, encourages people to pay attention to their feelings in the present moment, a skill often termed "mindfulness." Practicing mindfulness techniques within your yoga practice and then implementing them throughout the day can help combat stress over the long-term.

It Improves Sleep

Stress and sleep (or rather a lack thereof) is a vicious cycle. Stress can throw off your sleep, which, in turn, makes you even more stressed. Yoga can help break the cycle.

It Gets You Moving

Exercise is becoming increasingly popular among the medical community as a treatment for down-in-the-dumps symptoms such as stress and anxiety. However, high-intensity exercise can temporarily increase your cortisol levels, which may put your body (and perhaps even your mind) under additional stress, Gentle forms of yoga, however, use non-impact moves to help get the stress-relieving benefits of physical exercise without triggering the release of stress-related hormones.

YOGA FOOD TIPS AND ADVICES FOR GOOD HEALTH

☐Eat four times each day at four hour interims.

☐Never try to skip breakfast, it is the most imperative dinner of the day.

☐Never try to drink water with your feast – take water 30 minutes before a dinner.

☐When you eat a dinner, your stomach ought to be 1/2 loaded with nourishment, ¼ with water (taking 30 minutes before) and ¼ ought to be vacant for appropriate absorption.

☐Eat sustenance that is naturally cooked.

☐Never try to gorge or eat too less.

☐Nourishment ought to be delicious and simple to process.

☐Nourishment ought to be eaten with focus and in a quiet domain.

BENEFITS OF YOGA FOR THE MIND, BODY AND SPIRIT

☐All-round wellness. You are genuinely solid when you are physically fit as well as rationally and candidly adjusted. As Sri Ravi Shankar puts it, "Wellbeing is not an insignificant nonattendance of malady. It is a dynamic articulation of life – as far as how happy, adoring and eager you are." This is the place yoga helps: stances, pranayama (breathing systems) and contemplation are a comprehensive wellness bundle.

☐Weight loss. Yoga is advantageous. Sun Salutations and Kapal Bhati pranayama are some ways to help reducing in weight with yoga. Moreover, with regular rehearse of yoga, we tend to become more sensitive to the kind of food our body asks for and when. This also help keep a check on your weight.

☐Stress help. Little minutes of yoga amid the day can be of incredible approach to decreases stress that aggregates every day - both the body and brain. Yoga stances, pranayama and meditation are one of a kind procedures to alleviation stress.

☐Inner peace. We love to visit quiet, tranquil spots, rich in normal excellence. Little do we understand that peace can be discovered right inside us and we can take a smaller than usual get-away to experience this at whatever time of the day! Advantage from a little occasion each day with yoga and reflection. Yoga is likewise one of the most ideal approaches to quiet an exasperates mind.

☐Improved insusceptibility. Our framework is a consistent mix of the body, psyche and soul. An anomaly in the body influences the psyche and comparably offensiveness or fretfulness in the brain can show as a disease in the body. Yoga postures knead organs and strengthen muscles; breathing procedures and meditation discharge push and enhance insusceptibility.

☐ Better connections. Yoga can even enhance your association with your life partner, guardians, companions or friends and family! A psyche that is casual, upbeat and mollified is better ready to manage delicate relationship matters. Yoga and meditation chip away at keeping the brain cheerful and serene; advantage from the reinforced exceptional bond you impart to individuals near you.

Yoga is an amazing calorie burner and fat buster. It is particularly effective at fighting stubborn fat reserves that sneakily build up in your body after you reach the age of 40. Various studies conducted on the benefits of yoga have shown that yoga lowers the levels of various stress hormones, promotes insulin sensitivity, and augments your metabolic rate–all these changes work as signals to make your body burn fat at a faster rate.

Here are some wonderful and effective yoga poses that can help you lose weight easily, quickly, successfully, and in a healthy manner.

Anjaneyasana

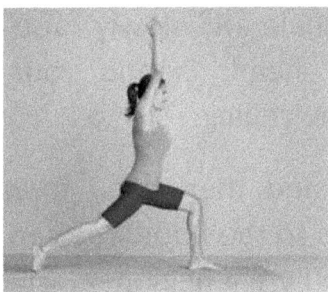

Also known as the crescent pose, Anjaneyasana is effective at firming your thighs, abs and hips, and losing the tough fat lodged in these parts. It fortifies your gluteus muscles, quadriceps, and your abdomen. It is excellent for relieving sciatica pain. Moreover, it expands your shoulders, lungs, and chest and enhances your stamina, concentration, core awareness, and balance. It is simple and easy to practice, which makes it perfect for beginners.

How to Perform It

1. To engagein this pose, stand straight with your feet together, arms at your sides, and toes forward.

2. Now, inhale and slowly raise your arms over your head. Extend your fingertips towards the ceiling.

3. Exhale and then bend forward. Bring your hands to the floor. You can bend your knees if you are a beginner.

4. Inhale and when you start exhaling, step your right leg backwards into the lunge pose. Keep your left knee bent to about 90 degrees. Inhale and gently raise your arms overhead and gaze forward. Maintain this pose for five to ten seconds and then return to the starting pose. Repeat these cycle five to ten times.

Virabhadrasana

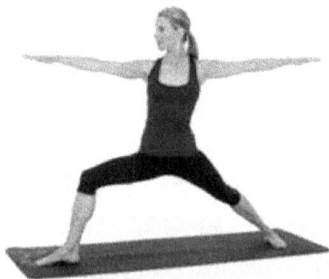

Warrior pose, or Virabhadrasana is an excellent yoga pose for stretching your back, strengthening your tummy, buttocks and thighs, and for losing annoying body fat. This pose is not suitable for people suffering from high blood pressure, back or knee pain, and any sort of condition pertinent to the limbs or joints.

How to Perform It

1. To execute the warrior pose, stand straight with both your feet together. Keep your hands by the sides.

2. Now, slowly extend the right leg a little forward and extend your left one backwards.

3. Bend the right knee gently, so you enter the lunge pose. Now, slowly twist your torso a little, so you face the bent right leg.

4. Turn the left foot sideways and exhale. Straighten both your arms and slowly raise

your body upwards and slightly away from the bent knee. Stretch the arms upwards.

5. Gently tilt the torso a little backwards to arch your back. Maintain this pose for ten seconds.

6. To exit the pose, exhale and then straighten the right knee. Push the right leg to return to the starting position. Be very gentle when exiting so you do not injure your legs.

Repeat it with the other leg. You can do it for ten minutes in the start and increase its duration with time. Watch this helpfulvideo to understand how to do this pose.

Surya Namaskar

Popularly known as sun salutation, surya namaskar is a series of different yoga Asanas carried out in succession. It has an amazing effect on weight loss as it makes use of lots of backward and forward bending Asanas that stretch and flex your spinal column, giving your entire body a profound stretch. This asana is a complete body workout that strengthens and works out every muscle in your body, promoting total body weight loss.

How to Perform It

Here's what you need to do to perform the sun salutation (images below)

1. Begin in the prayer pose or pranamasana. Stand straight with your feet together. Balance your body and weight on your feet. Open your chest and gently relax the shoulders. Inhale and lift your arms up. Now, exhale and gently bring forward your palms and unite them in front of your chest.

2. Next, get into the hasta Uttanasana or raised arms pose. Breathe in and lift your arms up and backwards. Keep your biceps close to your ears

3. Now perform hasta padasana or hand-to-foot pose. Breathe out and bend forward. Keep your spine erect. Slowly

bring your hands to the ground besides your feet.

4. After that, executethe ashwasanchalasana or equestrian pose. To do it, breathe in and push the right leg backwards. Bring your right knee towards the ground and then look upwards.

5. Next, perform the Dandasana or stick pose. To perform it, breathe in, and take your left leg backwards, straightening your entire body.

6. Now, perform the Ashtanganamaskara known as salutation with eight parts. Gently bring the knees down towards the floor. Start exhaling. Take your hips backwards and slide forward. Rest the chest and your chin on the ground. Raise your buttocks a little and arch them. Your hands, knees, feet, chin, and chest should touch the ground.

7. Next, perform the Bhujaangasana or cobra pose. Slide forward. Now, raise your chest upwards to form the cobra pose.

You can keep your elbows bent and shoulders slightly away from your ears.

8. After that, perform the Parvatasana, also known as the mountain pose. To do it, breathe out and lift your hips and your tailbone upwards. Maintain a V shaped posture.

9. Next, perform the equestrian pose, hasta padasana pose, and Hasta Uttanasana pose. We have described these poses above, so follow those guidelines to perform them.

10. End the sun salutation with the Tadasana pose. Exhale and straighten your body. Bring your arms down. Relax and analyze the various sensations taking place in your body.

Carry out these amazing poses and soon, you will experience a remarkable weight reduction.

Follow the image sequence below

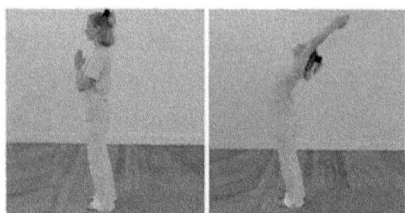

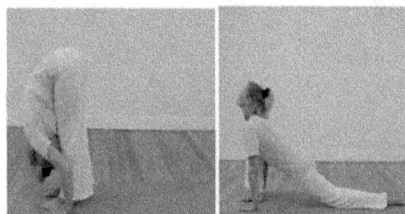

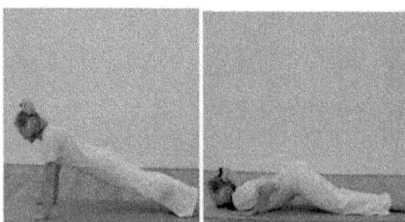

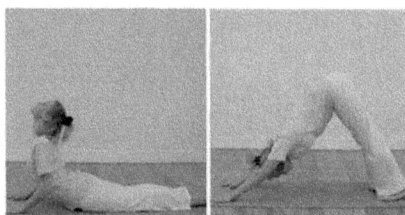

CHAPTER 14: THE BENEFITS OF YOGA

Yoga for the Body

Yoga poses encourage both strength and flexibility, but because the practice honors the person as a whole, you always work at your own pace. This is what makes yoga perfect for arthritis sufferers – you perform the poses within the boundaries of your own ability and comfort. When you're starting out, you might have some muscle groups that are weak, and that's fine. Gentle effort is all that's required to begin strengthening them. You'll also have stiff places you might not even be aware of, and it's a rare treat when you find a stretch that eases them.

For arthritis sufferers, the main benefits of yoga are improved strength, flexibility, and balance. Muscle strength is important because strong muscles can help to support and take strain off the joints. Flexibility in the joints will give you a better range of motion and improve your comfort, both when you're awake and when you're trying to sleep. And balance, largely a product of the first two, means you're less likely to suffer a painful injury that will take time to heal. All of these lead to an increase in mobility, and a reduction in pain.

So yoga soothes and fortifies the body, but there are a host of other ways it helps you. The practice has been shown to improve brain function, lower blood pressure, improve circulation, and build lung capacity. Many twisting poses aid digestion, and help with bloating and discomfort caused by the continued use of painkillers.

Inflammation causes or exacerbates many health problems, including types of arthritis. While short-term or sporadic yoga practice does not help with inflammation, there is some evidence that it can help, if you're dedicated. In 2010, Janice Kiecolt-Glaser, PhD, conducted a study at Ohio State University, Columbus. She measured the levels of proteins linked with inflammation in the blood of yoga practitioners. She found that newer participants had higher levels of these proteins than those who had been doing yoga for a while; however, there were no immediate changes in these levels in the short term. She notes that the people in her study were similar in terms of age, body type, and health habits.

Whether it was the poses, the exercise, the breathing techniques, or the meditation, it's encouraging to note that the participants also reported feeling better emotionally. Yoga will sometimes relieve the pain, but even if it doesn't entirely, it does help with your frame of mind. A good outlook has been shown to decrease your experience of the discomfort, and give you the fortitude to withstand it better.

As we've said, yoga brings us into touch with ourselves, body, mind, and spirit. It encourages self-care, and makes us more aware of how our bodies are feeling. This awareness can lead to a change in other habits as well, such as eating healthier, or getting more sleep. These things in turn contribute to your overall health, which reduces your pain and makes you stronger in both body and mind.

Yoga for the Mind

Yoga works on the nervous system, and it also stimulates our glands with its twisting and stretching. This is how it's able to help us feel more relaxed and at ease, reducing stress and anxiety and bringing emotional comfort as well as physical.

Part of the reason for this is that the slow, deliberate breathing techniques we use in yoga serve to distract us from the hundreds of trivial thoughts that run through our minds. When we pay closer attention to our inner self, we are able to think more clearly, and this makes us feel calmer. The more time we are able to spend in this calm state, the better able we are to detach from the external tensions affecting us.

Meditation has been shown to reduce stress, and this is especially important for people with arthritis and related conditions. Not only are you dealing with the regular problems of daily life, like bills, deadlines, appointments, and obligations, but you have an extra layer added by chronic pain. Now you're dealing with physical discomfort, loss of sleep and fatigue, physical limitations, job complications, and maybe even the loss of your independence and self-confidence.

Because of these extra physical, real-life challenges, it's especially important that people with arthritis pay particular attention to self-care, both physically and emotionally. Setting time aside for yoga will help you accomplish both.

Part of the challenge of dealing with anxiety is calming the body, because it is difficult to settle the mind when you're experiencing physical stress responses like shallow breathing, elevated heart rate, and sweating. Some people don't even realize when this is happening; they only know they feel terribly agitated. The regular practice of yoga teaches us to be self-aware and reach a state of calm more quickly and deliberately, through regulating the breath, and focusing the mind inward. Once the body begins to settle down, the mind can as well. As we have said, yoga addresses mind, body, and spirit as a whole.

Yoga and You

As you turn through the pages of this book, you may be inspired by the poses shown, but you may feel intimidated. Don't worry. These pictures are intended to show what your goal might be ultimately, but in almost every pose there are modifications, helpful hints, props, and exceptions for your situation.

Things you may want to have on hand:

A thick yoga mat

Yoga blocks

A yoga strap, or an improvised one like a scarf or belt

A thick pillow or two

A blanket you can fold into the desired shape

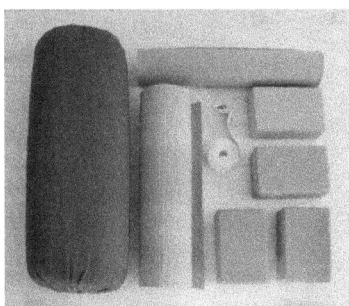

Read the instructions for the poses, and consider what your doctor or healthcare adviser has recommended. Try some of the easier poses first, always remembering to relax and breathe. The simple poses are stepping stones to the more demanding ones, and you'll be surprised how little time it takes to evolve once you've begun. You're going to feel so much better!

Some poses will feel awkward at first, and this is normal. You have not asked your body to do these things before, and even people without particular physical challenges feel strange when they begin. Do the poses the best you can, and soon you'll notice they're getting easier. Gradually, you'll build flexibility, strength, and balance.

It's natural to feel a stretch or a mild burn in your muscles, but you should never push a joint that's flaring. Any sharp pains are a signal to stop. And while you'll probably want some privacy to do your practice, keep safety in mind. Have plenty of props on hand to help you balance and do the poses. Most importantly, if your condition is severe, don't attempt difficult poses if there is nobody around to call to for help.

Are you ready to give it a try?

We can begin to form habits in as little as three weeks, and the yoga poses will start to help you even if you can only spare twenty minutes a day, starting out. What happens for many people is that they enjoy the practice so much that they stay with it longer, building more strength and flexibility, which in turn makes the practice more enjoyable.

So hop into something comfortable, take those socks off, and get started!

Chapter 15: What Is Yoga And How Can It Benefit Me?

The practice of yoga takes its roots far back into history. It is believed that the practice started in ancient India and made its way into the religions of Asia and the Middle East. Now the practice of yoga is worldwide, helping people to feel better physically and mentally. Yoga is not only a spiritual practice, but it includes your mind and body. Putting all of these elements together makes it possible to have a weight loss routine that will both clear your mind and relieve your stress.

In this society, many people struggle with maintaining a healthy weight due to stress in their lives. Speaking from experience, I find that I eat when I'm stressed out and tend to shut down physically and mentally. It has also been proven that stress inhibits your metabolism and immune system. Once I started on my yoga routine, I was able to focus on my stress and my body and create peace in my mind. I find that I no longer stress eat like I used to and that I have lost a significant amount of weight by having a regular yoga routine. Yoga is not just exercise. It is a way of acting and thinking that will help you to become healthier.

Essentially, yoga is the practice of using different poses and stretches while concentrating on your breathing and your body. While doing yoga, you are encouraged to focus only on what is going on in your body and let the outside worries of the world drift away. Meditating is also a part of yoga. Focusing on things that bring you peace and make you happy, you can help calm your mind. By having a total focus on your mind and body, you are able to control your breathing and your body. Each pose and stretch is meant to target a certain portion of the body, making it a great way to get physical as well as mental exercise.

The practice of yoga will help you become more disciplined in mind and body.The poses and exercises used in yoga call for you to move your body in certain ways while focusing on your "core" and your breathing.Essentially, you're focusing on multiple facets of your body at once, making it necessary to have complete control and concentration.If your focus is off, then your moves will be off balanced and shaky, making it difficult to achieve the goals of yoga.

Yoga can be performed by any person, whether they're an athlete or just beginning to exercise.The techniques of yoga go from basic to expert, and that makes it easier for most people to be able to perform them, no matter what their fitness level is.Whether you take a yoga class or watch an instructional video, the techniques are easily executed, making it a good all-around form of exercise.Depending on your skill level, there are different forms of yoga that can be used to fit your abilities.

No matter what type of yoga you choose to practice, there are many resources available to help you in your journey. This can range from going to the gym and taking a class to performing the moves with the aid of a video gaming system. Since it's a popular form of exercise and practice, there are numerous resources out there to fill your needs.

While there are many health and mental benefits to yoga, there are also emotional benefits. You will become happier and more in control of your emotions. By taking the time to learn about the practice and benefits, you are on the road to better physical and mental health. In the following chapters, I'm going to cover the types of poses that are useful for different areas of your life. Whether you want to focus on weight loss or mental awareness, yoga is a great practice to pursue.

Chapter 16: Is Your Lifestyle Making You Carry More Weight?

While we cannot completely blame our hectic, stressful lifestyle for our weight gain, it is largely a reason why we keep packing on those unwanted pounds. Constantly racing against the clock, not getting sufficient sleep and eating sketchy meals are the crucial reasons why we gain weight.When you sleep less, you generally eat more. When you sleep less, you are more stressed, and to beat that stress you eat more. Sadly you eat more of all the wrong things that are detrimental to the balance of your body. When you're rushing to meet deadlines all the time, you're missing meals or eating irregularly. You 'grab a bite' rather than sit down to a meal. When you eat in haste, you generally eat a lot more because you chew a lot less. Plus, when you eat in haste, you are generally eating fast food which is high in calories and does the most harm to your body. Perhaps it's time to stop and take stock of your lifestyle. Is it responsible for making you pack on the pounds? Are you getting enough sleep? Are you eating right? Are you getting enough time to de-stress? No?

Life will always throw stressful situations at you. You are constantly trying to accomplish something and you don't always reach your goals. You worry about your job, your kids, your responsibilities. You probably don't enjoy good quality sleep, and are not aware that bad quality sleep makes you wake up stressed and hungry.

Chronic stress leads to an increase in appetite and stress-induced weight gain. We need to look at our neuroendocrine system to understand this connection between our brains and our bodies. What helped our prehistoric ancestors to survive has become a threat to our lives because it causes weight gain. Basically, whenever we're faced with a stressful situation, a series of hormones are activated in our bodies. These include adrenalin, which gives us instant energy, corticotrophin releasing hormone (CRH) and cortisol which causes us to replenish energy through eating. Cortisol is the culprit that increases our appetites and prompts us to eat more.If we lived in prehistoric times this would be just fine, as we would have expended energy running from a predator and would need to replenish it through eating. We wouldn't be replenishing energy that our bodies don't require, and therefore our food wouldn't be sitting in our bodies, turning to fat, as it does now because we are not living in a prehistoric situation.

Let's look at de-stressing options. We would probably list television up front. Nobody would think that exercise could be a way to de-stress, but it is. However, there are some workouts that can be too vigorous, and therefore promote further stress rather than calm you down. The one practice that provides you with a total workout and promotes peace and calm is

Yoga – the discipline that ancient India lived by and passed down across generations; the holistic therapy to modern day stress that people across the world are turning to for solutions to their health problems and for weight loss.

Yoga as a discipline works from the inside out. By working on your chakras, it induces a state of calm and restful alertness that enables you to be more productive, and speeds up your metabolism so that you shed calories. When you are lighter in mind and elevated in soul, your body automatically responds, and becomes lighter...because you tend to require far less food to get through each day.Why do you require less food?Because whatever you eat is more efficiently processed and utilized in your body.

CHAPTER 17: YOGA POSES FOR ANXIETY AND PANIC ATTACKS

The yoga asanas on this section shall help you overcome anxiety and panic attacks:

Tree Pose

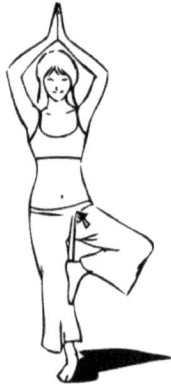

The tree pose can help you fight anxiety any day; however, getting comfortable with this pose is not always that easy. Follow the steps below to get the best from the tree pose:

How to go about the tree pose:

Stand erect, lift your right foot up, and place your toes on the floor. Turn out your right knee to the right. Focus your gaze on a particular point and repeat the same pose on your left side using your left foot.

Once comfortable with that first step, place the sole of your right foot on your left ankle, turn out your right knee to your right side, focus your gaze on one point, and repeat the pose on your left side.

Once comfortable with your foot on your ankle, try balancing the sole of your right foot on the side of your left calf muscle, and repeat this pose on your left, hold and practice deep breathing.

Cow Pose

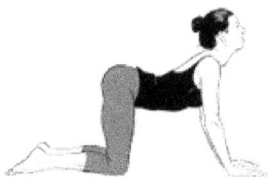

The cow pose is one other yoga pose that can help you manage anxiety. :

How to go about the cow pose:

Get down on all fours. Keep your knees set directly below your hips and keep your wrists, elbows, and shoulders perpendicular to the floor. Keep your head centered in a very neutral position and fix your gaze on the floor.

As you breathe in deeply, lift your chest and sitting bones toward the ceiling while allowing your belly to sink in the direction of the floor. Then lift your head to gaze forward.

Exhale and return to the all fours position. You can repeat this pose about 10 times.

Camel Pose

The camel pose makes it possible to experience deep spinal extension without any need to support your weight using your arms. This is a flexibility pose you can do anywhere to help you reduce anxiety.

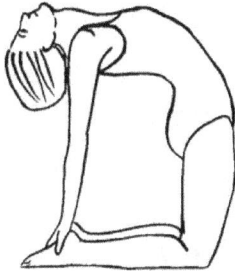

How to go about the Carmel Pose:

Kneel on your yoga mat with the knees placed a hip width apart and the thighs forming a 90% angle to the floor. Slightly spin your thighs inward while narrowing your hip points. Keep your buttocks firm, but not hardened. Keep your outer thighs soft while pressing your shins and the tops of your two feet into the floor behind the mat.

Keep your hands resting at the back of your pelvic region with the base of your palms on top of your buttocks and fingers pointing downwards. Press your front thighs backwards to stop your front groins from puffing forward. Inhale deeply and lift your heart by keeping your shoulder blades pressed against your back ribs

Now lean against your firm tailbone and shoulder blades. Keep your head up and your chin near your sternum. Your hands should remain on your pelvis

Make sure your lower front ribs do not protrude sharply in an upward position because this will harden your belly and compress your lower back. Release your front ribs and lift the front of your pelvis in the direction of your ribs, and then lift your lower ribs away from your pelvic region to keep your lower spine lengthened.

Firmly press your palms against your heels, with the bases of your palms pointing in the direction of your toes. Turn your arms externally to allow your elbow creases face the forward direction. Your neck can remain in a neutral position, neither extended nor flexed. You can also drop your head backwards.

Hold this pose for 30-60 seconds. To release, draw your hands to be at your hip points. Inhale deeply as you lift your head and torso upwards by pushing your hip points downwards towards the floor. Then rest in the child's pose and draw a few deep breaths.

Chapter 18: How To Practice Yin Yoga

It is essential to know how to practice as well as what to practice. These pointers will guide you into a better practice. It is quite natural for all of us to push ourselves beyond our limits to get an Asana perfect. We forget the basic concepts of a yoga practice. We actually contort our bodies to meet the requirements of a particular posture. But, when practiced the right way – according to the ground rules – all forms of yoga practices gift you the physical benefits while offering a sense of inner peace. All we have to do is to be mindful by setting an intention and paying attention.

Let's take a deeper look at this...

The Basics

"Having seated (himself) in ... a room and free from all anxieties, (the student) should practice yoga, as instructed by his guru," says Hatha Yoga Pradipika.

And, for this to happen, we need to follow certain other factors... Here are those!

Setting an intention

Setting an intention boosts the impacts of the benefits we receive from the practice. It could be physiological, emotional, psychological, or spiritual. When an intention is set before a Yin Yoga session, it sets the stage for an increased flow or energy by removing the blockages.

The intention behind our practice determines the ideal time for our practice.

When to practice Yin Yoga?

We can practice this style of Yoga

☐When our muscles are relaxed so that the stress in the connective tissues are still

☐Early in the morning to ease the stiffness

☐Late in the evening or minutes before bed to calm the mind and stressed muscles

☐ As a stretching session before a Yang practice

☐ After a Yang yoga session to render a meditative touch to the practice

☐ When you feel fatigued for better energy

☐ To restore Yin-Yang balance in our lives

☐ To energize ourselves after a long trip

☐ During menstrual cycle (for a woman) and postnatal care to conserve and nourish energies

While we can practice Yin after a sitting for a long time, it is better to avoid it during winters after prolonged sitting. In such a state, the body turns stiff and refuses to oblige.

In the end, the right time is when our minds and bodies say yes. So, it better to ask the body and mind whether it is ready for the practice before we begin one.

How often should you practice Yin?

Even though Yin Yoga helps to balance our Yang energies, it is advisable to adjust the duration to meet the body-mind requirements. We can practice daily for about 20 minutes to calm the hyper Yang. Alternatively, we can allow yourself to indulge in a 90 minute long Yin Yoga practice to soothe our roaring mind.

Teachers often advise starting with just once a week. We can slowly evolve the practice according to your needs. Getting in touch with our bodies and minds will give us a clear idea about how to move forward. As we age, incorporating more Yin Yoga sessions in our life will nurture the joints and bones, helping us stay healthier.

Tips For Better Practice

Here are certain general rules that could help us enjoy a Yin Yoga practice in a better way.

Since Yin Yoga focuses on deep breathing, it is advisable to avoid loading ourselves with perfumes.

Practicing on a relatively empty stomach is wise. Hence, we should aim to eat something light at least 2 hours before the practice.

If you are planning to practice Yin Yoga during mornings, give yourself at least half an hour after waking up to restore the natural elasticity of the muscles. Empty the bladder and bowels before the practice. If possible, take a refreshing shower.

Wear loose, comfortable, and breathable clothing that is generous on the body.

Keep props handy. Straps, blocks, cushions, and blankets are ideal as they would help us make the most out of the forward bends and reclining postures.

Turn off the phones. If you do not have a dedicated space, make sure that you inform your family beforehand. Just like meditation, tranquility and silence are essential to make a Yin Yoga session successful.

☐Remove bracelets, wristwatches, glasses, jewelry, or any such thing that could hinder the practice.

☐Light a few candles and spray some essential oil elixir in the air to set the tone for the practice.

A word of caution

Certain poses need extra caution. So, if you have any injury, recent or old, or any other health conditions, please do consult with your physician before your begin your tryst with Yin Yoga.

If you are pregnant or have any cardiovascular conditions, it is advisable to practice under personal supervision to make the most out of practice.

Stick to a gentle, short practice if you feel over exhausted.

These are the basic things we should know before we start the practice. Now that we have talked about the theoretical side of Yin Yoga let's prepare us to experiment with some postures and flow in the next two chapters.

Are you ready to enjoy a beautiful journey?

Yoga is a category of physical and mental exercises that aim to improve strength, flexibility and overall wellbeing. Yoga is well-known for postures, which are specific movements and bodily positions that test flexibility, stamina, balance and strength. Another prominent aspect of yoga is the focus it places upon improving and regulating breathing. The practice of yoga is believed to have originated in India over 5000 years ago, yet it is continuing to evolve as other countries and cultures develop and adjust yoga's paradigm. Yoga is associated with Hinduism, with the core yogic teachings originating from the Upanishads or ancient Hindu spiritual texts.

The scientific literature on yoga is still in its nascent stages. However, it is generally agreed upon by the scientific community that yoga does improve balance, flexibility and strength and has little risk of injury.

There is also a body of research to suggest that yoga can help tackle stress and depression and reduce overall bodily pain.

Even though yoga is often classified as a type of exercise, it is not considered to be a particularly taxing or difficult type of exercise. Therefore if you are trying to burn calories or improve your level of fitness, other forms of activity may be more effective. Nonetheless, yoga is effective at improving overall musculature, especially in the older individuals, who may struggle with or be vulnerable to injury with other forms of exercise.

Most notably, yoga is well documented to strengthen the ankles and knees, which reduces the chances of falling, which is a notable risk for the elderly. On top of this, yoga is less strenuous for people with arthritis than other forms of exercise, which overall helps it be a fantastic choice for older adults.

Another fantastic aspect of yoga is its gentle learning curve. Yoga is a rewarding activity for people of all abilities; whether you are already fit and strong and looking for a challenge, or whether you need to start at the very beginning.

It is important to note that there are dozens of different types of yoga, which vary dramatically in their practices. Some types of yoga are mostly esoteric, predominantly focusing on spiritual and mental release. Other types of yoga are closer to a dance workout or music routine, aimed at appealing to a modern demographic who want to burn fat. Therefore if you try a school or type of yoga and find it isn't to your tastes, don't be disheartened; there is bound to be a type of category that is tailored for your needs.

Although it is possible to self-teach yoga, it is wise if at some point in your journey, you join a class or yoga community. As with any form of exercise, there is a risk of injury, especially if your technique and form is poor. Joining a class with a certified teacher allows for someone to point out your mistakes and reduce the chance of straining your body. Additionally, working with other people is a well-tested way to improve motivation & discipline.

CHAPTER 20: THE HISTORY OF YOGA

Yoga is about much more than getting into a few odd looking poses and holding them for a few seconds; the history behind the discipline is quite rich and interesting, and the benefits you receive from those poses are very far-reaching too!

Yoga found its first beginnings around 5000 years ago in India. At this point the discipline wasn't really recognized for its exercise properties, but was more about helping the flow of energy, or chi, through the body. As you can see, yoga is about the spiritual side of things too.

The actual solid facts about its beginnings are a little sketchy, because the original scripts were not really written in a way which was meant to be preserved! Having said that however, the way yoga has moved on and developed can be traced to a large degree. Most yoga enthusiasts cut yoga down into four main developmental eras.

- Pre-classical yoga

- Classical yoga

- Post-classical yoga

- Modern period

This is basically how yoga has developed from its original state, into what it is today. Obviously nowadays yoga is much more commercial than it has ever been, and it has lost a lot of its spirituality in some ways, focusing more on exercise, but those who take the time to learn about it in fullness will be able to learn a lot about the 'other' side of yoga.

Basically, pre-classical yoga is its most purest form. This was when yoga was founded, by the Indus-Sarasvati tribes in Northern India. You will see the first mentionings of yoga in the Rig Veda, a set of sacred writings which consisted of songs, rituals, and mantras which were used by Vedic priests. From this we can gather that yoga was originally developed not to help bring about flexibility and health benefits, but rather to invoke a higher wisdom, attract good karma, and open up the mind to help solve problems.

Obviously nowadays we use yoga as beneficial aid for our health, but it's certainly worth keeping in mind the more mystical side of it. For instance, how much do you know about chi, chakras, and namaste?

Let's check these out one by one.

What Are Chakras?

Everyone has heard of chakras, but not everyone really know what they are. Chakras are opened up by practicing yoga, and this then allows the clear flow of energy throughout the body. Each chakra is set to a certain part of your life, e.g. confidence, self-awareness, the ability to love etc. If you have a blocked chakra then you will be experiencing a problem in that particular part of your life, the area which the blocked chakra pertains to.

Yes, it does sound a little complicated, but once you familiarize yourself with what each chakra is, and once you learn more about it, as your yoga hobby progresses, you'll see just how truth this whole principle is.

These are the chakras which are present in the human body:

• Muladhara / Root chakra – This chakra is linked to feeling grounded, the importance of family, and a sense of belonging.

• Svadhisthana / Pelvic chakra – This talks about fertility, basically about the health and functioning of your sexual organs, but can also be linked to creativity and ideas/new beginnings.

• Manipura / Naval chakra – This is one of the most important chakras in the modern day because it is linked to a sense of self-esteem and confidence. This is an area which many people find a blockage in, and you will find many yoga classes concentrate on this particular chakra in particular. The naval chakra is also about productivity.

• Anahata / Heart chakra – As the name would suggest, this particular chakra is about your ability to open your heart to love, accept and give, and to forgive.

• Vishuddha / Throat chakra – This particular chakra is about telling the truth, but it is also about speaking what is on your mind too.

• Anja / Third eye – This is one of the two most important chakras (along with the one we'll speak about next), and guides the rest of the chakras to work correctly. Linked with your higher self and your inner voice (intuition), this is a chakra which many people meditate on.

• Sahasrara / Crown chakra – Along with Anja, this is one of the higher chakras, and that is also in the sense of where it is located; Sahasrara is located above your head. This particular chakra is about spirituality, psychic ability, and learning/accepting who you are on the inside.

If you feel that you have a problem with any of the areas mentioned in this chakra descriptions then you can give yourself a helping hand by learning to meditate and focusing on that particular chakra. Meditation isn't as hard as it might seem, but it does take practice. For instance, if you find that you are having an issue forgiving someone and it is causing you to feel bad or toxic on the inside, you may have a blockage in the Anahata (heart) chakra. Therefore meditating on this chakra can help clear the blockage and allow energy (chi) to run much smoother.

Simple Meditation

So, we've talked about chakras and we've mentioned that you can help clear blockages and problems in your life by using meditation to work with these chakras. How does this tie in with yoga? Well, yoga, chakras, meditation, and spirituality are all linked together, so learning how to work with the whole package will help you develop your yoga habit overall much more comprehensively. Yes, you can use yoga simply as an exercise tool, but you're really missing some of the interesting stuff if you only do that!

Okay, so you are probably aware that meditation is difficult. Yes, it is difficult, but with practice it can be done. The most difficult part of learning to meditate it understanding how to turn off the noise inside your head and outside. We live in such busy times, there is always noise of some kind, and our heads are running through the million tasks we need to do that day. It's no wonder that we feel stressed out and burnt out by the end of each day.

Learning to turn off the noise is the key to meditation, so you need to find a quiet spot which allows you to give this whole meditation thing a go.

Try this:

• Dedicate a certain time per day to your meditation. This needs to be a time which is totally free, e.g. perhaps at the end of the day or beginning; it's no good trying to stuff this time in-between other appointments because you won't be able to clear your head very effectively.

• Find a location where you won't be interrupted. Your bedroom is a good place, or your living room when no-one else is in the house. This needs to be somewhere you feel comfortable, and somewhere you can make yourself comfortable too, e.g. with cushions or blankets.

• Turn off your phone, or at least put it on silent. Listening out for a vibrating phone call or a 'ping' message from someone is not going to put you in the best frame of mind to meditate. You need to turn off the outside world for the short amount of time you're going to be focusing on yourself.

• Sit in a comfortable position. You don't have to sit with your legs crossed like you would imagine, but if you find that a comfortable position then go for it! You can sit in an armchair, you can lay down; basically, find out what works for you – meditation is a totally personal kind of deal.

• Close your eyes and focus on your breathing. Breath in through your nose slowly, pause for a couple of seconds, and then exhale through your mouth slowly too. Turn your whole attention to your breathing, and imagine your cares and aches being exhaled along with your breath. You will find that this process helps calm your breathing down, it helps you feel more relaxed, and it may even make you feel a little sleepy too!

• If any thoughts come into your mind, don't get stressed about it, simply acknowledge them and allow them to float back out of your mind just as easily as they entered it. This is the part which most people find the most difficult, because once a thought pops into your head, you're likely to dwell on it and try and think it through – stop yourself! There's plenty of time for overanalyzing your life later on!

• Starting at the tips of your toes, scan your body for any aches, pains, or discomfort. When you spot some discomfort, imagine the pain being exhaled with your breath. Work up your body until you reach the top of your head. You will find that this whole process takes your mind away from anything else.

• Once you have scanned your body, take some time to think about how you now feel – you should be feeling totally chilled out and almost floating. Acknowledge that feeling. Focus back on your breath.

• Slowly bring yourself back to the present.

This whole process can take anything from ten minutes to an hour, it's totally up to you, but it's important not to rush things, because meditation is not something you can just cram in between daily tasks!

Give it a go, but don't beat yourself up if you stumble a few times – meditation takes time and practice. We mentioned meditating on the certain chakras, and that is something you can build up to once you have mastered the art of tuning out the noise inside your head and in the outside world. To meditate on a chakra you may use crystals, or you simply may use visualization techniques, imagining how you think that particular crystal would look, it's color etc.

What is Namaste?

If you go to a yoga class you might find that you hear the word 'namaste' quite often. At first you'll probably be a little confused and wonder what it is you're being asked to do, but the truth is that you're not being asked to do anything, it's simply a greeting, a 'thank you'.

Namaste has its roots in the Sanskrit language, and loosely means 'I bow to you'. At the end of a class you may find that your teacher says this whilst placing his or her hands in a praying position in front of the heart chakra and their head. You are expected to return the favor and repeat what they have just done.

What does it mean?

It basically means 'well done', and it is a form of congratulations, a thank you for your hard work. Yoga is a karmic kind of deal, so when someone says something pleasant to you, you are expected to return it to keep the flow of energy positive and up lifting.

The Difference Between Yoga and Pilates

You will hear these two disciplines mentioned in the same breath a lot of the time, but it's important to realize the differences. Basically, yoga is about encouraging and improving flexibility in the muscles and joints, whilst also relieving stress and anxiety at the same time, by focusing on breath. Now, pilates on the other hand is a little more heavy going than yoga is, and basically focuses on the ability to relax the muscles, strengthening them at the same time.

The two disciplines are very similar in some ways, but it's important to identify which one is best for you. If you are new to it all, yoga is probably the best place to start, because this will introduce you slowly to this whole world, encouraging that flexibility that you will need, in order to reap the many health benefits.

This has been a lengthy chapter, one which will have given you a lot of information to digest and think about. Whilst we haven't talked yet about how to do yoga, it's important to know about its history and background, in order to really understand what it is you're doing. For instance, if you simply jump straight into a yoga class, you won't have the first clue why you're doing something, and when your teacher mentions the various chakras, you won't have any idea what they're talking about. From reading this chapter, you know have a basic knowledge to build on.

In our coming chapters we will get much more practical in terms of actually getting into yoga. First things first however, we need to talk about the different types of yoga available. There are many to choose from, and some suit beginners, some suit everyone, and some suit advanced ability levels. Our next chapter will introduce you to these various types of yoga, and will allow you to pick the right one for you.

Chapter 21: Common Mistakes To Avoid

Before registering for one of the most effective yoga vacations in 2013, you should be ready to ask yourself is how much you need to know about yoga? A lot of people who begin yoga feature energy and nonsense into learning how to perform like acrobats! That's the primary mistake they make. You can find numerous topics on what to study within this exercise, both on a real one plus an emotional level as well. You, therefore, need to avoid the following through your yoga sessions.

Driving the human body too far

As a beginner, your body is not used to these kinds of workouts, and when you start them, to avoid any damage, it is essential to consider this. That doesn't suggest you have to follow along with every single thing they are teaching. Your teacher should be advised of any new client in a class to steer him/her through the exercise independently. Some poses might appear easy, and you'll seek them out, and then realize that you are currently straining other parts of your body. Do not be tempted to test any new complex poses by yourself.

Absence of balance and awareness throughout the program

Complete focus is needed by yoga! Meditation about the hand does not mean thinking too much or hard about anything. Use small attempt to enter a peaceful state of mind and you must have a mind that is comfortable.

Yoga features a means of releasing anxiety through particular pressure points on your body. This could require you to create in ways that may stress one other side. Therefore, you need to balance every exercise you are doing throughout the procedure. Failure to this, such tension may lead to interior injury to your muscles or joints, which have a lot of relaxation and time to heel. Simply relax!

Keeping your breath for too long

Yoga may contain some hard exercises! This doesn't imply any energetic workouts; it is the method that you cause and also the interval you are forced to stay for. People forget to breathe and concentrate more on the cause as this happens! This may cause absence of oxygen in some elements of your body just like the brain, that leads to fainting during yoga or passing out. Constantly advise the coach instead of trying out poses that could trigger more damage than good for your body if the procedure is becoming complicated. This is a justification why you need an instructor by doing a yoga teacher education evaluation.

Conclusion

A mudra is a seal, something that creates an impression, and it is also the impression itself. A mudra is a seal in the form of a hand gesture, containing and evoking meaning. When you make a mudra, then, you are both creating and receiving information. Each mudra has a particular function and symbolism, so when you make a particular mudra, you seal that information and purpose into your body and your consciousness.

Do you want to experience peace? To access your inner energy? To experience reverence? To connect to the world around you? To make a commitment? Begin with a mudra.

Mudras are easy to perform anytime, although sitting in the lotus position and focusing on the healing can be an advantage. Although mudras can be used for healing certain ailments, regular practise of mudras will contribute to your overall good health and can be used as a preventive measure. Continuous practice of the mudras will create minute changes in your body using pulse centres on parts of your hands, which trigger certain healing processes within the corresponding body part

You can create mudras at any time and in any place. A beautiful way to begin a regular mudra practice is to start and end your day with one. Try holding a mudra for a few minutes, experiencing what the mudra feels like and contemplating its meaning. If you sit to meditate, try creating the mudra at the beginning and at the end of your practice.

Just as you form an asana with your body and are then formed by the experience, you shape a mudra with your hands and are consequently shaped by it. When you arrange your hands in any mudra, you seal a specific impression into your consciousness. Your body and mind can and will shift as a result of a regular mudra practice. You become the artist and the artwork, the creator and the created.

www.ingramcontent.com/pod-product-compliance
Lightning Source LLC
Chambersburg PA
CBHW051729020426
42333CB00014B/1220